THE

Multiple Sclerosis

"[A]n important book for patients and their families. It includes resources for travel, MS organizations, employment laws, alternative and complementary therapies, and medications."

— *Newsday*

"Blackstone is an ideal person to write about the first year of living with MS . . . [she] delivers a truthful but 'don't panic' picture of MS, validating and informing about the facts, the fears, and the nuts and bolts of living through each day fully and intelligently."

— *InsideMS*

"Ms. Blackstone provides the newly diagnosed with love and comfort and helps them face their fears in a reassuring way that is filled with hope. I wish my family knew of such a book when we found out my mother had multiple sclerosis over twenty-five years ago."

— GRIFFIN DUNNE

MARGARET BLACKSTONE is a graduate of Yale University. She was awarded the Murray Fellowship and wrote and translated poetry in Mexico for a year. She is the author of several books on a variety of medical topics, including *Beat Diabetes* and *Recovering from a C-Section,* a poet, and an award-winning author of children's books. She lives in Greenwich Village with her son.

ALSO BY MARGARET BLACKSTONE

Beat Diabetes
Recovering from a C-Section
Girl Stuff
The Egg White Cookbook

THE COMPLETE FIRST YEAR® SERIES

THE FIRST YEAR®

Multiple Sclerosis

An Essential Guide for the Newly Diagnosed

Second Edition, Completely
Revised and Updated

Margaret Blackstone

Foreword by Saud A. Sadiq, MD

MARLOWE & COMPANY ■ NEW YORK

THE FIRST YEAR®—MULTIPLE SCLEROSIS, *Second Edition*:
An Essential Guide for the Newly Diagnosed

Copyright © 2003, 2007 by Margaret Blackstone
Foreword copyright © 2003, 2007 by Saud A. Sadiq, M.D.

Published by
Marlowe & Company
An Imprint of Avalon Publishing Group, Incorporated
245 West 17th Street, 11th Floor
New York, NY 10011

AVALON
publishing group incorporated

The First Year® and A Patient-Expert Walks You Through Everything
You Need to Learn and Do® are trademarks of
the Avalon Publishing Group, Inc.

The Library of Congress has cataloged the previous edition as follows:
Blackstone, Margaret.
 The first year—multiple sclerosis : an essential guide for the newly
diagnosed / by Margaret Blackstone.
  p. cm.
 Includes bibliographical references and index.
 ISBN 1-56924-522-3
 1. Multiple sclerosis—Popular works. I. Title: Multiple sclerosis. II.
Title.

 RC377 .B627 2002
 362.1'96834—dc21

ISBN: 978-1-56924-261-2
ISBN-10: 1-56924-261-5

                                              2002141436

9 8 7 6 5 4 3 2 1

Designed by Pauline Neuwirth,
 Neuwirth and Associates, Inc.

Printed in the United States of America

For Lucrezia Funghini and Mary Conley,
Friends beyond measure,
For Trent Duffy,
another inestimable friend,
And in memory of Lenny Dunne

"GREAT NECESSITIES
BRING FORTH GREAT VIRTUES."
—ABIGAIL ADAMS

Contents

Foreword

by Saud A. Sadiq, MD

MULTIPLE SCLEROSIS is a disease that is potentially disabling, physically and psychologically. Frequently it first strikes in early adulthood at a time when a person is at his or her physical prime. To be told "you have multiple sclerosis" leads to a numbing vulnerability that is often psychologically devastating. After they learn of the many treatments that are available today and are reassured by their physicians, some patients can start "living again." However, many others experience a gamut of emotions ranging from depression, despair, and anxiety, to anger and hostility.

One of the most effective treatments for all the negative connotations associated with a diagnosis of MS is the support of one's peers. Patients are usually most assured by the experiences of other people who are in the same boat. In a similar vein, my new patients often ask for literature about available treatments and simply about how to cope.

Margaret Blackstone, the author of this valuable book, is a patient of mine. When I first told Meg of her diagnosis, I could see that her bewilderment and uncertainty about her future were blotting out almost everything else I told her that day. In the next few visits, as she regained her equilibrium, she asked me where she could find guidance about managing her life. At that time, there was little written for patients that I could recommend to her.

Now Ms. Blackstone, an experienced medical writer herself, has rectified that situation. This outstanding book is an answer to her many questions about MS and much more. It is intended to be used by a patient from the day that he or she is diagnosed and will help enormously in getting the patient back on an even keel. At the end of the first year the newly diagnosed patient will be able to appreciate that MS is being conquered. There is a real revolution going on in therapies for MS and the future looks better every year. This book is part of that future.

When a patient is diagnosed with MS there are two parts that have to be considered. One is MS the disease. The other is the affected *individual*—the patient. No two patients are identical, and I have found that in treating patients a doctor should always be cognizant of the individual. Meg's book is fully grounded in her experience, but it also gives guidelines for all of those living with MS in the first year. It provides newly diagnosed patients with much information and comfort that I think they will find extremely helpful.

Meg, the patient and the writer, is having a conversation with other patients. Even though they have their own disease and issues, they will find much here that will help them first cope—and then overcome—MS.

As an MS specialist, I feel that new patients will benefit from reading this book because it offers a wealth of information on the disease and it helps new patients understand and participate in their treatment programs. In addition, this book will help new patients understand their emotional reactions to the diagnosis and offers practical advice on how to cope with these reactions.

In the years since Meg wrote *The First Year—Multiple Sclerosis,* I have found that many if not most of my new patients have already obtained this book and appreciated how much help it gave them, recommending it to me for other patients. My staff tells me the same thing. We also recommend it to those few new patients who have not read it, and they are very grateful.

In this revised and updated edition, Meg adds even more new and important material for first-year patients, and any and all patients coping with MS, including new research information, the latest news on Tysabri, the newest disease-modifying treatment, and also information about the new technologies in testing, treating, and coping with MS. I don't know of any other book that does so much to both instruct and comfort those who are newly diagnosed with MS.

Meg's book is an important one for patients, their loved ones, and also for doctors who treat those with MS. It is superbly written and meets a yet unfilled need for all of those newly diagnosed with MS.

—Saud A. Sadiq, MD
Director, International Multiple Sclerosis Management
Practice and Multiple Sclerosis Center of New York

Preface to the Second Edition

THIS REVISED edition of *The First Year—Multiple Sclerosis* adds to the extensive investigation and interviewing I did for the original book and expands upon my ongoing experience with tests, treatment, and life regimen. You'll also find an updated guide to treatment options, new information on alternative medicine and MS, as well as information on results of the most recent clinical trials on treatments for and possible causes of MS, and an update on risk factors for MS. I've visited again with many of those whom I interviewed for the first edition and, wherever such information is of interest, briefly updated you on how I'm doing (in two words, very well!).

What I have found most helpful in reviewing all the research for this new edition is realizing how much more is astir regarding MS in the medical community, particularly regarding what really causes MS, new, more effective treatment programs, and what might finally provide the cure for MS.

Perhaps the most important lesson I've learned as I move forward living with MS is not to try to stay the same, be the same, act the same—instead, the point is to let MS change you and in the process to make sure you let it change you *for the better,* which it will if you try and if you let it. As one newly diagnosed person told me, "I refuse to live without joy in my life." I couldn't agree more. Think of this as a new beginning and you will already have won your first battle.

— Margaret Blackstone,
September 2006

Introduction

EVER SINCE human beings recognized that they had minds, the workings of our consciousness have confounded writers, artists, scientists, philosophers, psychiatrists, and all the rest of us. Many medical conditions that directly affect the brain and the central nervous system have challenged and fascinated all those who treat these conditions, as well as those who suffer from and manage them.

Multiple sclerosis is one such perplexing neurological disease. Not only is it one of the most complex human conditions to understand and treat, but it's also one of the most variable diseases, affecting each of us in very different, individual ways and to varying degrees. Much is still not known about how it affects those it strikes, or about how and why episodes of symptoms are triggered.

Now that you have been diagnosed with multiple sclerosis, you will do best if you are in the care of a specialist in multiple sclerosis, and if, at the same time, you educate yourself about your disease and learn how to manage it. The more you are in control of your world and your grip on the disease and the course it may take, the greater sense of emotional security you will achieve and the more stable your day-to-day life will become.

I know. I have multiple sclerosis, and I live with it and manage it well.

What happened to me

The first inkling something was wrong was somewhat more than an inkling. One February evening in 2000, I fell straight down the stairs in my house and landed at the bottom with an aching bum and a gash in the back of my head that was bleeding. Once the gash stopped bleeding, I knew enough, from my experience as a medical writer, to stay awake for three hours to ensure that I did not have a concussion. In the morning, my pillow was stained with blood, I was a bundle of aches and pains, and there was a psychedelic eggplant of a bruise blooming across my bottom, but otherwise I was okay—except for the dizziness.

That feeling persisted, so after a few days, I called my doctor. He found nothing in a neurological exam, but sent me for an MRI, just in case. I went for the test by myself and I waited more than an hour. The radiology center was short-staffed, and I was more annoyed than I was nervous.

Luckily, it turned out that I'm one of those people who aren't bothered by MRIs. During the test, I kept my eyes shut and thought of the children's book I was in the middle of writing. It was a very productive forty minutes.

On Friday afternoon, a week later, I went to a funky lamp store with my son to pick out a light fixture that we needed. There was a light blinking on the answering machine when we got home. It was my doctor. His words are etched indelibly in my memory. "Well, you don't have post-concussive syndrome, but you do have multiple neurological abnormalities." I called his office right away, but it was almost five o'clock, and he was already gone. I couldn't reach him all weekend, though he had told me to call him. I lived through Saturday and Sunday, not knowing what was going to happen next. On Monday morning, after taking my son to school, I went about getting a duplicate set of films and finding another doctor. Illness is one thing. Uncertainty is one thing. Mistreatment is another.

It would be my new doctor who presented me officially with the diagnosis of multiple sclerosis (MS). In fact, I learned, I had a variety of the disease called relapsing-remitting MS.

Some people choose a quest; others have a quest thrust upon them. Like it or not, that was the beginning of my quest. I use the word "quest" deliberately, since multiple sclerosis is as much a mystery as it is a disease. I decided from the very beginning to be the best sleuth I could be in discovering the clues that would lead me to the best doctors, the right treatment, and as many positive outcomes on this journey as possible. I might never catch the culprit—the cause of MS is still unknown—but I would find the best way to cope with MS in my life.

This book is the result of a year of investigations, consultations, tests, and treatment. It may not solve the mystery you face with MS, but it will illuminate healthy and productive ways of managing your life and help you chart your best individual course.

Nobody knows what the future holds. Those of us with MS are simply more intimately acquainted with this tremendous uncertainty. What we can do is help to modify the course of our disease in many ways, no matter what stage of disease or disability we have when we are diagnosed. To make a lousy, but accurate pun, none of us is immune. We are in it together, sisters and brothers in the mystery of MS.

Groucho Marx once declared that he would never join a club that would want him as a member. Groucho had nothing on us. Although we might also refuse to join any club that would have us, this club doesn't listen. This club doesn't take members. It drafts soldiers. It's up to us to rise to the occasion. This book will help prepare you.

How to use this book

You are right to be shocked by your diagnosis. Shock is a human response that allows the mind to accept the unacceptable gradually, from a psychological distance, rather than being overwhelmed. When you recover from your first wave of shock, the next shock might be caused by a realization of just how much you need to absorb about this chronic illness. To make the realization process more palatable, I've tried not to overwhelm you with too much information in the chapters that involve the first days and weeks in which you are learning to cope with your diagnosis. I have also tried to be sensitive to the emotional component involved in managing MS well, since how you manage stress is an important factor in coping with the disease.

The structure of the book reflects that concern. Each chapter is divided into two sections, Living and Learning. The Living portion is geared to help you manage how the disease affects your daily life, relationships, and overall mood. The Learning portion gives you the hard facts that you need to know to manage the disease well in every way. Needless to say, given the sometimes amorphous nature of MS, these sections may overlap. But that's not at all bad, since how you manage your disease depends on integrating living and learning as you go along.

The format of the book—day to day for the first week, week to week for the rest of the first month, and month to month thereafter—is meant to make it easier for you to absorb the information you need as you need it, and at a pace that works for you. The last thing you need right now is something else that's hard to understand and make sense of. For instance, in the first days, I try to give you the information you must have to begin coping well with MS, without giving you too many facts to digest (those come later), and to provide you with ways to manage the practical and emotional issues you will confront early on.

Given the variety of symptoms, the mysterious origins of MS, and the quixotic nature of the course it takes for each of us, I need to state that if you are beginning to read this book because you have been diagnosed during a severe episode and have yet to start treatment with one of the disease-modifying drugs, it is okay to skip ahead to the section on medication before you read earlier portions of the book.

I would also like to express thoughts of hope and encouragement to those of you who have had a more severe introduction to living with MS than others of us. Even if you're off to a difficult start, don't despair that the disease will not get better. One of the men I interviewed, Paul, was diagnosed almost ten years ago after vision problems and a sudden fall out of bed one morning. Within days Paul's left side was almost paralyzed. He then began treatment with one of the disease-modifying medications. As of this writing, he is in better shape than when he was first diagnosed. He holds the same executive position, is still enjoying a happy family life with his wife and children, experiences no numbness or paralysis, and walks with a cane only now and then. I repeat: only now and then. May a similar success story belong to each of us in our own way!

I would like to add, however, that just as MS affects each of us individually, so are we each unique in how and when we want to hear or read, digest, and accept all the information that we will eventually need in order to live well with this disease. Some of us want more and want it all at once. Some of us want less and want to let it in a little more slowly. Feel free to browse the table of contents and move to the day, week, or month where you feel you need more information now. For example, if you are an absolute fanatic about diet, you might jump ahead to Month 3 to learn how to customize your diet to suit your condition as well as possible.

To keep things as simple as possible for the newly diagnosed reader, all medical terms that appear in **boldface** in the text are defined in the glossary at the end of the book.

I will not prescribe

In living with multiple sclerosis and researching this book, I've compiled a great deal of important and varied information on the condition known as multiple sclerosis that can be of service to you as you begin to make the tough and necessary decisions about your course of treatment. However, even though I am a professional medical writer, I am not an M.D. or a nurse-practitioner and have no business prescribing any course of treatment.

On that subject, I want to make clear that I do understand one great difficulty all of us MS patients face: the level of symptom aggravation and disability we display is so variable that it can prevent us from identifying and sympathizing with one another. I know that I am very lucky to be walking and to have only four lesions in the myelin cells within the brain. I have extraordinary respect for those who cope with more symptoms and attacks and who even endure disability early on.

I hope that others who have been diagnosed with MS will gain courage from reading this book, but I do not, in any way, proclaim that there is a single set of recommendations that ensures success in coping with MS. I will give you information about MS, tips that have helped me and others deal with daily life during the first year, the inspiration I feel we all need to have when dealing with MS, and the sense of determination that will keep us all coping, and coping well. In short, I want to be of benefit to all who read this book, even though the course that multiple sclerosis takes is as variable as human personality.

Rather than being prescriptive, this book is meant to make you aware of all the options and to be an aid in your decision-making process. It will also provide important information to help you deal with insurance issues and other financial matters. Once you have finished reading it, you will have the knowledge you need to understand your disease, and the treatment options and creative ideas for improving the quality of your life on a day-to-day basis will be available to you, so that *you can make your own informed choices.*

Where the focus is

The idea behind this book is that the better you manage this disease in the first year after your diagnosis, the better your chances will be for managing it well in the future and avoiding any major disabilities. This assumes that you are a person who wants to and will take an active role in managing your disease and its symptoms.

Because the course of MS is so variable and so confusing at times, once again, you should feel free to turn to the section you need most at the time. For example, some of us enter the process of diagnosis with visible symptoms that need to be managed. If this is true for you, turn to the learning section that deals with managing symptoms. If you are young and married and very much want to have a family, but wonder what the consequences may be, not only for your baby, but also in terms of your disease, turn to the living section that deals with planning and having a family.

The more you know about MS, the more accurately you can ask the questions you need to ask and describe the symptoms and episodes that affect you—and thus get the help you need. For practical reasons, the more information you have, the more you will be able to participate in and guide the course of your treatment.

Keep on learning

I think the best thing your first year of living with MS can do for you is to inspire you to keep on learning more about your condition and how to manage it even more creatively and productively.

I hope that you will use the resources mentioned in this book to keep up on research into treatments and into alleviating symptoms. You may also want to talk to others with MS as you become more and more comfortable with realizing that the course of the disease is different for everyone, and that everyone has something to contribute in terms of how to cope. Another option is to become involved with your local chapter of the National Multiple Sclerosis Society (NMSS) or visit their website. The NMSS has a very active research department peopled with doctors and other health workers dedicated to treating and curing MS.

Since MS is one of the most provocative medical mysteries, this fact should add to your inspiration to learn more and keep informed on new treatment developments and new efforts toward a cure. After all, you may be able to do your part in delivering more clues that lead to important answers. You may enter a clinical trial, or decide to do a family history and a personal history of trauma and infection in your childhood and teenage years that you may share with your specialist to add evidence to support studies on what the origins of the disease may be.

Another way to keep learning is to return to this book as a source and a resource, now and then. Sometimes, we can't take everything in all in one reading, and if you revisit a section of this book a second, or even a third time, you might find something there that you don't remember from your first reading. In addition, you may want to use the suggestions for additional reading recommended in the chapters and in the recommended reading list provided at the end of the book.

The best resource for continued learning and understanding is yourself and your reliance on yourself and those you love. The best way to keep on learning is to live every day as well as you can and allow yourself to accept new experiences with an open heart and mind, and a new appreciation of the challenges and rewards your life presents.

THE FIRST YEAR®

Multiple Sclerosis

An Essential Guide for the Newly Diagnosed

Reeling

ALL TRAUMAS were not created equal, but all traumas hold one thing in common. Trauma is like the tides. The waves roll in and roll out again, only to roll back in once more. You will manage these first days and weeks and months living with MS much more smoothly once you begin to accept the waves of feelings you will inevitably experience. Consider this the tides of adjustment.

First shock, then fear, and then you become overwhelmed. You may get so overwhelmed that you feel mentally unsteady, as if you're reeling. A mixture of these emotions makes for a rough few hours, whether it took your team of doctors six months to diagnose your MS or you were struck by a severe episode that made the presence of MS suddenly incontrovertible. Some people float above their diagnosis—shock actually can make this a possibility. Some panic. Some weep. Some accept it in stony silence and fall apart later.

All of these responses are normal, and you should not feel embarrassed or weak, or blame yourself for any of your reactions. They are your reactions and feeling them and accepting them will help you in your all-important new goals to minimize the stresses in your life and manage the stresses you must inevitably endure both creatively and constructively.

To a person, all of the women and men I interviewed with MS expressed the belief that what was most helpful in the early days was to take in the news little by little, bit by bit, to avoid the nearly unbearable paralysis that comes with being overwhelmed. Go as slowly as you have to, and remember it's okay if lack of acceptance and denial are part of your period of adjustment, as long as you do not hide from the truth forever. For instance, Pamela, who is now in her late thirties, spent a long time in denial: "When I was first diagnosed, I panicked and so decided it wasn't true. I was in my late twenties and couldn't allow myself to believe the diagnosis or even the idea of having MS to be part of my life. I lived for many years ignoring **symptoms**. Then I grew up and went to a neurologist. I was diagnosed again, and this time I didn't panic. Now, whenever I regret not facing the truth sooner, I remind myself that what I am able to deal with now, I couldn't deal with then."

Accepting the truth, one realization at a time, is your right and will probably stand your health in good stead during this undeniably trying time.

What's going on with your body

All of us with MS have many things in common, but one big difference probably is how we were first physically and medically introduced to our condition.

For many of us, an acute attack led the way to an almost immediate diagnosis. This will cause a certain personality type relief. He or she may sigh and say, "Finally, I know what's going on. Now, let's get on with it." For others, there may be anguish, panic, and moments of fear and feeling sorry for oneself. In either case, however, you are lucky in one respect. With an exact diagnosis, you have one less mystery to cope with and can now get on with coping with the mysterious ways of MS.

For others, the road to diagnosis was much longer; it may have taken years and included odd symptoms erroneously construed to mean anything from perimenopause to Epstein-Barr virus. You wondered what was going on with your limbs, head, speech, and sight. The causes of your clumsiness, fatigue, or buckling knee remained a mystery. Only after having a battery of tests, including the MRI and spinal tap, and all other possibilities ruled out, were you handed the diagnosis of MS.

I had this latter kind of experience. I endured five months of uncertainty—is it this? Is it that? Is it something worse than this or that? In an important way, I was relieved, finally, to have a concrete diagnosis. By the time my specialist, Dr. Saud Sadiq, uttered that one sentence—"You have MS"—I'd already spent enough time in the room with fear and in the church of self-pity to say, "Okay, let's get to work." Now I had a target to aim at—hitting the bull's-eye of living well with MS.

All the innovative medications available and all the first-rate doctors in the world won't do as much good as they will if you bring your good attitude and your great sense of humor to this first year and every rewarding year to come. Therefore, the most important thing to say to yourself is: My life isn't over, a new stage is just beginning. Let's get on with it.

IN A SENTENCE:

It is normal to feel shock when diagnosed with MS, and coping well with the disease depends on accepting this and then moving forward.

learning

Beginning to Understand MS

LIKE IT or not, no one can tell you exactly what MS is or where it comes from. Even the experts don't know precisely what MS is or why it has stricken you. While MS can be clinically diagnosed, it is a disease composed of variables. Most of the doctors who specialize in MS will tell you they, too, are in the midst of researching one of the true mysteries of the medical community.

What we do know is that multiple sclerosis is a disease of the **central nervous system (CNS)**. The cells of the CNS, which includes the brain and the spinal cord, are covered with a protective **myelin** sheath. In people with MS, three abnormal processes begin to occur in these cells.

1. Patches of inflammation begin to occur in areas of the brain and spinal cord.
2. The myelin sheaths around the cells affected by the inflammation begin to deteriorate. This is called **demyelination**.
3. The nerve fibers, or **axons**, stripped of protective myelin, begin to be destroyed. They lose the synapse connection

that these myelin sheaths ordinarily provide. Without the ability to conduct these signals, the CNS cannot communicate the vital information that it is responsible for conveying to the rest of the body. As a result of this miscommunication within the body, a person will exhibit symptoms of MS.

It's extremely important to understand that this process of demyelination and deterioration differs from person to person and that the course of the disease may also vary greatly.

The damage to nerve cells in the CNS is believed to be caused by what might be called a confusion in an individual's immune system. In other words, instead of becoming activated by an invading virus or infection, the immune system turns on itself and begins to attack the nerve cells. When an individual's immune system backfires or turns against the very organs and tissues that it is meant to protect, the condition is classified as an **autoimmune disease**.

In MS, when the cells of the immune system go on the attack, they attack the healthy cells of the CNS and destroy the myelin coating that protects individual cells, leaving scar tissue in place of the healthy cell. These demyelinated areas, also known as **plaque**, appear as tiny white patches on an MRI and indicate the existence of a neurological abnormality, in this case, MS.

Signs and symptoms

Symptoms are the complaints that a patient will explain to the doctor during the medical examination, such as a feeling of fatigue or having balance problems. **Signs** are what the doctor will discover during the examination. The most common signs for MS are instances of sensory disturbances, overactive reflexes, vision disorders, weakness in specific limbs, and abnormal patterns of speech. Whereas symptoms are expressed in everyday language, signs are terms that medical professionals understand, and that laypeople rarely use. Together, symptoms and signs are termed *findings*.

While all the symptoms of MS are distressing, some may cause more trouble than others. For example, if you have had problems seeing, you will need help from your doctor. You do not have to think, however, that this is your future, since many people with MS do not experience severe enough symptoms to restrict their normal activity.

The principal symptoms of multiple sclerosis are:

○ Fatigue, experienced in a variety of ways (an overall sensation of exhaustion for no apparent reason; tiredness after strenuous exertion, exercise, or a long day, etc.).

○ Weakness, experienced as leg buckling or simply lack of strength in the limbs and hands.

○ **Spasticity**, a term used to describe when an arm or a leg feels tight and its movement is slower and less smooth. Spasticity may also be experienced as involuntary movements of the limbs due to increased reflexes.

○ "Tight band" sensations, experienced as a girdle-like band around the trunk or the lower legs.

○ Numbness, experienced as a sudden lack of sensation, much like the feeling of a limb "falling asleep," or as cold feet.

○ Issues of vision, experienced as double vision, a sudden, temporary loss of sight in one or both eyes, and/or a central blind spot in one or both eyes.

○ Issues of gait and balance, experienced as a hesitation in the limbs while walking and a continual sense of being off balance.

○ Urinary incontinence, experienced as a frequent need to urinate, including some leakage.

○ **Vertigo**, experienced as the room spinning and/or objects that are still appearing to be in motion.

○ Pain, experienced as sharp, shooting sensations and electrical spasms that seem to occur inside the limbs rather than on the skin, though skin sensitivity may also cause pain.

No one with MS experiences all of these symptoms. If you do have a symptom, make a note of it and tell your doctor at your next consultation.

Hard Facts

THERE ARE about 400,000 people in the United States with multiple sclerosis.
About 2.5 million people in the world have multiple sclerosis.

Each week, more than 200 people throughout the world are newly diagnosed. This number will only increase as the testing methods used to diagnose MS become even more refined and accurate.

Of all those who have been diagnosed:

○ 75 percent will remain ambulatory throughout their lifetime and will never need a wheelchair.

○ 40 percent will not experience symptoms that are debilitating enough to limit their normal activity.

○ 20 percent will experience a benign course of the disease, one that does little or nothing to disrupt their lives.

The life expectancy of MS patients has increased by more than ten years since the 1950s.

The role of stress

Multiple sclerosis is intimately related to how you manage the stress in your life. Flare-ups are more likely to happen when you are stressed. Even as you grapple with the immediate need to learn about MS, you also need to learn how to moderate the amount of stress in your life and to master productive ways of managing the portion that is unavoidable.

Your first task in stress management is staring you right in the face—managing the stress of being diagnosed with MS. As I have mentioned, detailed information about the possible causes and effects of the disease is presented throughout this book. Don't try to digest it all at once; instead, you may want to pick and choose *what* you read and *when* you read it. The truth is, you can probably obtain all the information about MS that you'll need *for now* during one visit with your doctor.

If questions do come up that nag at you and cause anxiety, write them down first and then call your doctor's office. That way, you're not at a loss for words when you speak to a nurse or your doctor.

You'll want to become your own "stress referee," working to keep much stress at bay. Here are some things MS patients have found helpful just after being diagnosed:

○ Relax. Go for a long walk, listen to music, or watch your favorite comedy on video or DVD.

○ If possible, take another sick day from work. Give yourself a chance to regroup emotionally.

○ Meditate. In its simplest form, meditation means calming your nerves and helping yourself relax and gain some emotional distance from your anxieties.

○ Let your answering machine screen your calls. Your friends and family naturally want to express their sympathy and many of them will have opinions and advice. It can be overwhelming to talk with everybody right now, so return phone calls when you feel up to it.

The notion of having multiple sclerosis, that mystery of diseases, is scary. Even as you begin to incorporate your diagnosis into the existing fabric of your life, it's important not to inundate yourself with too much information at once. An overload of advice and knowledge can cause stress, taxing your immune system by upsetting you more and wearing you out.

IN A SENTENCE:

> MS is an autoimmune disease that begins when the immune system triggers the destruction of the protective myelin in the cells of the central nervous system.

Reeling Back In

HOW PEOPLE respond to their diagnosis is as variable as
an individual's symptoms. You may want to get a grip on yourself right now; you may be in a state of semi-shock; you may
even still be crying or hysterical; and certainly you may be (and
probably are) exhausted. All of these are natural, reasonable
responses. But it's time to at least get yourself ready to do the
best for yourself. This will help you maintain a strong grip on
managing your treatment once treatment begins.

There are unspoken rules in our culture regarding how we
cope with the diagnosis of a serious illness. We are supposed to
cope with it bravely and with absolute aplomb. This is unrealistic. Not only is the diagnosis of MS overwhelming at first, but
people often find themselves swamped by strong emotions.
Feelings of grief, anger, self-pity, fear, depression, and others
compete for attention and make it hard to concentrate on anything else. Instead of maintaining a stiff upper lip, as society
might prefer, it is okay to spend some time now examining how
you feel.

The diagnosis and the grieving process

The degree of feelings of loss and sorrow that accompany your initial diagnosis will vary from person to person. But whatever your particular sense of loss might be, consider it normal and natural. Indeed, going through some degree of grieving is part of a healthy adjustment process.

The fact is, you must begin to balance a paradox. You think, "Yes, I am the same person I was yesterday," and yet you also ask, "Where is that person I was yesterday? Today, I am a different person." The first thought is a sort of healthy denial; the second is a sign of acceptance. Both of these feelings are elements of the stages of grief, which were first delineated by Elisabeth Kübler-Ross in *On Death and Dying*.

As with mourning any other experience of an important loss, don't expect an orderly progression of emotions. Allow yourself to experience these different moods as they come and go. Eventually you will move past grief into facing the ordinary challenges of leading an active, satisfying life.

Feeling sorry for yourself

It is natural and even necessary to feel your own very private moments of despair. How you manage these times of reflection and doubt will make a difference in your overall outlook. Even with self-pity, there are good ways to go about it.

Here's what you should not do: Walk down the street cursing everyone who's eating fast food, talking on a cell phone, or living heedlessly. Ask yourself, "Why not him? . . . Look at all these people. They're young and overweight and they don't take care of themselves. . . . How can she act as if she doesn't have a care in the world? . . . How come they're healthy, and I'm not?"

It should be clear that such thoughts are mere conjecture, not truth. In addition, everyone in the world has problems, even if they're not glaringly evident, and, over the course of a lifetime, everyone faces one health challenge or another.

The best way to cope with your life challenge is not to compare it to those of others. Look at the trees and the view, not the others on your street struggling with their own problems.

There are better methods to help you through feelings of self-pity. Put the lights on low or light a candle and listen to Bach's Brandenburg Concertos or another beautiful work; then sit quietly, crying a few tears if you must, or writing sad musings. Or, if you are athletically inclined, take a long jog or stroll, and run or walk those blues out of your head and heart. Another method to cave into and get beyond your justifiable sadness is to curl up in bed, hugging a pillow if your partner is not available, and have a good cry.

If you're not the type to feel sorry for yourself alone, call a true friend. Lean on his or her shoulder in person, or you can even have a good cry over the phone.

Any of these indulgences will turn out not to be indulgent at all. They act as a form of rest or exercise and so will increase your strength and stamina, which increases your ability to reel yourself back in from the shock of the diagnosis.

Dealing with anger

Many people get angry when they are diagnosed with MS. This is reasonable, but you will not want to live with this anger for long. Anger expressed is anger completed, but silent anger festers and grows into resentment. If you let your anger fester, you will eventually take it out on yourself or those you love. So you have to find ways to manage your anger, before it makes you sick or causes you to lash out at your loved ones.

If you are the physical type, you might release your anger through a good workout a few times a week. If you belong to a gym, try the punching bag. It's fun, and it's very satisfying when you're angry. But physical exercise alone will not tame the beast of anger at your own fate. You'll need to talk about your anger to understand it and place it behind you. Try to talk through the bad blow fate has dealt with family, friends, and your doctor. If that is not enough, consult a therapist.

In fact, it's possible to manage your anger and turn it toward constructive use. For instance, it can motivate you to begin an exercise program or to learn to give yourself your own injection in order to remain self-sufficient and independent.

Getting your rest and a good night's sleep

Given the news you've been dealing with, and the swirl of emotions competing for your attention, chances are you didn't have a good sleep last night. Brenda, a thirty-year-old woman, said she felt terrible after she was diagnosed. "I was also exhausted by the time I finally was given the news, which only made it harder to bear up."

As you set out to establish a healthy relationship between yourself and your MS, it is vital to ensure reasonably good sleep habits. A lack of sleep can exacerbate your symptoms, so sleep is your first defense against the fatigue of MS. In addition to getting enough sleep, you will also want to add short rest periods to your routine. Lie down and close your eyes for a few minutes. If you are afraid of falling asleep and napping for too long, set an alarm. A short rest can rejuvenate you for the rest of the day and leave you relaxed and less anxious, which will allow you to fall asleep more easily at night.

During the early days of coming to terms with your diagnosis and formulating a treatment plan, you should take extra precautions to try to get a good night's sleep. Here are a few pointers that have worked for some with MS.

- Monitor your caffeine intake. Avoid coffee or other caffeinated beverages in the afternoon or at dinner.
- Make exercise part of your daily routine. Being physically tired can help an overworked brain succumb graciously to sleep. (However, don't exercise just prior to going to bed, or you may be overstimulated and unable to court sleep.)
- Drink plenty of water during the day, but taper off in the evening to avoid trips to the bathroom during the night.
- Restrict your intake of alcohol to one drink. Too much alcohol can and will disturb your sleep. (Alcohol also can cause or exacerbate depression, and short-term depression is a common consequence of a diagnosis of MS.)
- Drink an herbal tea before bedtime (but don't drink too much!) while reading or listening to music.

○ If you enjoy a bath, take a tepid to warm bath (forget hot baths; extremes of temperature may exacerbate symptoms of MS) with your favorite bath salts an hour before retiring.

○ For those interested in herbal remedies, valerian root can be a calmative before bed. (Of course, check with your doctor first.)

If sleep continues to elude you, or if you find yourself waking frequently and having difficulty falling back to sleep, talk to your internist or MS specialist. Your doctor will be able to prescribe something for sleep that is safe and nonaddictive. If you are experiencing pain, such as from a sense of stiffening in your legs, I've found that two extra-strength ibuprofen not only help to relieve the pain, but also make me drowsy enough to dose off.

You might even try some of the effective over-the-counter remedies. My doctor recommended Benadryl. The antihistamine causes drowsiness and even helps you return to sleep should you wake in the night. For the first few weeks I relied on the antihistamine to help me get to sleep. Now I take it only when I find I'm having trouble getting to sleep.

IN A SENTENCE:

Accepting all the various feelings you are having about your diagnosis is preferable to denying them and thus being unable to move on.

learning

Tests

GIVEN THE quirky nature of the course that MS may take, you may already have had many tests before hearing your diagnosis. But if you've picked up this book because your doctor has mentioned MS as a possibility, he or she may be sending you for a series of tests right now. Because MS is such a hard disease to define, most doctors are very cautious about making a diagnosis and they want to rule out all other potential conditions before making a definitive pronouncement. This valid caution can result in your having to have more than a single MRI and office medical examination.

In case you're facing more tests, then, here's a look at what's involved for the common procedures used in helping to determine an MS diagnosis.

Magnetic resonance imaging

Magnetic resonance imaging (MRI) is the gold standard for neurological diagnoses as well as for spinal-cord injuries and other conditions. What an MRI does for those of us being examined for positive proof of the demyelination caused by MS is to simplify the process of identification. An MRI can identify even the smallest area of demyelination or plaque, differentiating such locales from a tumor or blood-vessel damage due to an injury. This makes the job of your doctor much simpler and your diagnostic process much easier. One study of the test's efficacy showed that 96 percent of those people diagnosed with MS had abnormalities on their MRIs.

A nurse or physician's assistant will get you ready for your MRI. You lie down as comfortably as possible on a gurney-like table. In most cases, you will be provided with a set of headphones to muffle the sound of the machine as it is X-raying your brain or spinal cord. Then the table is pushed into the MRI chamber, where you are enveloped in darkness in a tiny tunnel for the test. Most MRIs take approximately forty-five minutes and consist of three or four series of X-rays with a pause lasting a minute or two between each series.

If you have claustrophobia or if you are anxious, an MRI can be somewhat traumatic. Ask your doctor to prescribe an anti-anxiety medication and take it an hour or so prior to your appointment. You'll be glad you did.

Just before you enter the chamber, close your eyes and do not open them until you emerge after the MRI. Not seeing how closely confined you are can help keep you from becoming claustrophobic.

Spinal fluid examination

A spinal tap, or lumbar puncture, is 85 percent effective in establishing that the abnormalities in the spinal fluid may strongly indicate MS and only MS. In cases that are difficult to diagnose, examination of the spinal fluid is also used to rule out what you do *not* have, such as Lyme disease, HIV infection, or syphilis.

Cerebrospinal fluid, or spinal fluid, is a clear fluid that bathes the spinal cord and brain; it provides a protective, shock-absorbent environment for the sensitive central nervous system. Changes that occur in the CNS due to disease may be reflected in the spinal fluid.

In cases of multiple sclerosis, **myelin basic proteins**, which are associated with the myelin in the CNS, are usually elevated in the spinal fluid. Other proteins, called **antibodies** or immunoglobulins, that are associated with MS may also be elevated.

The test is performed by inserting a needle into the area around the base of the spinal cord and extracting some spinal fluid. The test is very safe, and the body replaces the fluid quickly. However, you may want to request a prescription for a painkiller, since headaches are a common side effect of the test.

Other tests

MRIs and spinal taps are the most common tests used to confirm MS. Some neurologists and hospitals also still employ other tests.

Computer tomography. Computer tomography of the brain, commonly known as a CT scan, uses X-rays to create a whole picture of the brain. Different areas in the brain have different densities. The computer used in a CT scan analyzes the absorption of X-rays by these areas to create the image of the brain.

Before a CT scan is performed, you will be injected with a contrast material, a fluid that circulates throughout the blood vessels in the brain. The opacity of the liquid helps to illuminate parts of the brain that contain numerous blood vessels. In terms of MS, a CT scan does not give the same amount of visual detail as an MRI, so flare-ups and even large areas of demyelination may be too small to be seen. Still, for the time being, CT scans are often utilized during the process of diagnosing MS.

Electroencephalography. An electroencephalograph, or EEG, measures electrical activity in the outermost layers of the brain. This is also referred to as brain wave activity, but this test cannot show damage to structures deeper in the brain.

Evoked potentials. Evoked potential studies involve exposing a person to specific stimuli. Such stimuli include flashing lights, the shifting checkerboard pattern produced on a computer screen, clicking noises, and small electrical shocks. I've had them all, and these tests are not risky. They are easy to tolerate, although the one with the small electrical shocks, which measures the level of numbness, is no picnic. It doesn't hurt, but it is highly disconcerting.

The clicking noises produce auditory changes. This test is called a brainstem auditory evoked potential.

The shifting checkerboard pattern is a test that creates a visual evoked potential. This test can make you dizzy, so sit still for a few minutes when you are finished.

Flicker-fusion tests. Flicker-fusion tests are not used as frequently as other diagnostic tests in sorting out whether or not a person has MS, but some doctors find them helpful. The test is considered psychophysical and is used to assess a person's ability to discern the flickering of a small red light. The light is made to flicker rapidly, and in the case of a person with MS, it will often tend to blend into one beam of light, as the flicker becomes indiscernible to the affected eye.

IN A SENTENCE:

Because MS is such a confusing condition, you may face further tests to eliminate other possible illnesses before you are given a definitive diagnosis.

DAY 3

Whom Do I Tell?
What Do I Say?

AS YOU'RE adjusting to your diagnosis, and dealing with the amount of feelings that it's brought up—whether denial, fear, depression, anger, grief, or any number of emotions—the last thing you probably want to do now is tell others who are close to you the news. Sharing the news with your immediate family, extended family, friends, and loved ones can be extremely difficult, especially when you are still getting used to the idea yourself. Even as you crave their sympathy and you want to count on their support, you may dread their reaction or have mixed feelings about taking them into your confidence.

It's natural to have mixed feelings about telling others you have MS. Keep in mind that whom you tell, and when, is all up to you. There is no set way to go about this, so trust your instinct and do what is comfortable for you. Many people start with their immediate family, so in this chapter we'll discuss telling your spouse or partner, your children, and, if you're single, your boyfriend or girlfriend. Telling your parents and friends is discussed in Day 5 Living, and discussing your MS at your workplace is the subject of Day 6 Living.

Your spouse or partner

Your husband, wife, or live-in partner will usually know what you are going through as you are taking the tests that lead to a diagnosis. However, if, for whatever reason, you never said anything while you were being tested, now is the time to share the news.

When Sally was telling her husband, she tried starting with a joke. "I said to him, 'Honey, I have something to tell you, and no, I'm not pregnant. My doctor thinks I may have MS.' Then I took a deep breath. He was quiet for a second, but then he said, 'What do we have to do?' I was relieved and touched—bowled over by his response, in fact."

If the response you receive is similarly loving and supportive, be grateful. No one else can be as great a source of emotional and physical support as your spouse or partner. Share this book, and encourage him or her to learn about the condition you're facing.

Sometimes, however, a partner seems unable to accept the news, especially if you show no visible signs of MS. He or she prefers to remain in the seemingly safe haven of denial. For instance, my husband initially refused to believe me when I told him I had MS. Try not to be too disappointed if your partner does this. It's a natural reaction, one that is generally prompted by love for you and fears about your health, and you should try not to be hurt by it.

If this happens to you, make an appointment with your MS specialist or internist for the two of you. Explain ahead of time to the doctor that you need some assistance in helping your spouse face the news. Usually, this does the trick (my MS specialist communicated all the facts in a comforting, rational way, so my husband could accept the diagnosis).

If you continue to have trouble convincing your partner of your new health status and of your need for both emotional and sometimes physical support, you might want to consider couple's therapy.

Telling your children

After Ben told his wife that he had MS, they agreed he would wait until the weekend to tell their sons himself, so they would have time to digest the news. "Our boys are eight and ten, so I didn't give them all the gory details. I just said, 'Hey, I have this new thing. It's called MS. It's a condition that may make me tired and give me other symptoms. At least it explains why I was having all that eye trouble.'

"They both asked me if I was okay. I was so touched I almost choked up, but I saved that for later.

"Then I said, 'Please don't go looking it up online. You'll find all sorts of spooky stuff that may not necessarily happen. If you do go online or tell kids at school and hear stuff about MS, promise me you'll come to me and tell me about it.' They promised. Of course, the older one couldn't resist the temptation. Thank god, at least, he told me. One evening he searched the Web and came to me saying, 'Dad, are you going to end up in a wheelchair?' I said, 'Listen, if I end up in a wheelchair it'll be because I'm ninety and I've just gotten too lazy to walk anymore.' So far as I know, he's cured his need to know more, at least for now." One has to admire both Ben's son's honesty and Ben's attitude. Keep in mind that your children will find out. Therefore, you might as well be the one to tell them.

When and how you tell your children will test the mettle of your parenting. Some parents make too much of what they have to tell. Others make too little of it. And there are those who don't tell at all—until symptoms or hospitalizations make the diagnosis impossible to conceal.

In the beginning, when you are going through tests and procedures and don't have any definitive diagnosis, not saying anything more than that you have a couple of doctor's appointments is a sensible option. For teenagers, however, it may not suffice; you may want to have a casual family meeting in which you explain simply that you're going through some medical tests that are going to take up time and emotional energy, and ask the family to cut you a little slack until you know what's going on.

Once you have a definitive diagnosis, the situation changes. Now is the time to say something. Some parents recently diagnosed with MS have consulted a family therapist to help frame what has to be said in the clearest and least disturbing way possible.

If you are inclined not to tell at all, there are both emotional and practical reasons why this may not be the best approach. Not telling is hard on the whole family, including you yourself. A comfortable home environment is a blessing in coping with this chronic condition, but by keeping your MS a secret from your children, you add to the stress that you face. Your kids may not know *what* is going on, but they can feel and sense that something is out of the ordinary. Kids also have very creative imaginations, and without knowing the facts, they may let their young minds go wild with wondering and anxiety.

There are countless practical reasons to share the news with your children. Your treatment may involve injections you give yourself at home, often followed by a need to rest. Your symptoms could flare up in front of your kids (for instance, while driving your children to soccer practice, you could have a vision episode and have to pull over to the side of the road). Your fatigue could sweep over you on the evening of the school play or another event your child will find it hard to accept that you've missed.

My son's pediatrician told me, "Tell the truth, but don't tell too much." My boy was ten at the time, and this was excellent advice to follow. If you're unsure about it, speak to your MS specialist or your child's pediatrician, and discuss the pros and cons with your spouse or partner. (If you are a single parent, all of the same advice applies.)

If you do sit down to tell your children about your diagnosis, try to get the big information on the table without having to go into details that might confuse them or lead to further questions. Depending on the age of your children, their reactions and questions will of course vary.

The first question on a child's mind when confronted with a parent's serious illness is frequently "Will you die?" The answer is no. Keep in mind that "No" is a complete sentence, and saying it decisively will do wonders to help your child accept the news.

When your young child asks if the disease is catching, once again the answer is a concise no. All that your child wants to know is that MS is not like chicken pox or pinkeye—you can't catch it. Older children may wonder if they are at risk. The added genetic risk is about 1 percent, but until your child is old enough to search the Web for this information, it's reasonable and honest to say, "No. We don't know who gets MS or why, but just because I have it, doesn't mean you'll get it."

Even if your children are old enough to hear that, as yet, there is no cure for MS, tell them about the disease-modifying treatments that slow the course and sometimes can stabilize the disease. Here, it's important to answer with a resounding yes. Since all of these treatments involve injections (except Tysabri, which is administered intravenously every four weeks; see Week 2 Learning: Your Treatment Options), your children will be able to accept the idea of Mom's or Dad's needing a shot a lot easier when they realize just how much this medication will help you to remain active and healthy. If you are asked whether the shot hurts, you might want to fudge a bit and explain that at first it did, but now you are used to it.

Finally, particularly with young children, it is important to reassure your children that your relationship with them has not changed and will not change. You may want to reassure them that you will still be their parent, always and no matter what.

Other living situations

Since not everyone who gets MS is in a first marriage with kids, let's look at the situations of those in so-called nontraditional families.

If you live with a roommate, the roommate is bound to suspect something is wrong when you are on the phone with doctors, going to numerous doctor's appointments, and carting around unwieldy MRIs to obtain a second opinion. It may be in your best interest to reveal what is going on in order to relieve tension and avoid having a roommate start to conjecture the very worst.

If you are divorced and have told your children, whatever your relationship with your "ex" is, it will probably be easier in the end to share the information briefly and frankly with your children's other parent. My divorce from my son's father was fraught with all the inevitable arguing, anger, and trauma, yet we do a decent job of coparenting and have forged a new, if delicate friendship over the past few years. I never thought twice about calling him up and telling him that I had MS and that I had told our son but not told him too much. We rarely talk about it, although sometimes he surprises me by asking me how I'm feeling.

If your estrangement from your ex-partner is extremely difficult, you might want to wait to tell him or her and your children as well. Your children should not be given the burden of carrying a secret from their other parent—and if they're younger, they may not be able to keep it at all.

If a previous marriage ended in divorce but was childless, there is no need to relay the information. If you get along, you may simply want to.

Telling your boyfriend or girlfriend

The young person who is dating and is diagnosed with MS has a special situation. What the relationship is going to become has not been determined, and now this monkey wrench has been thrown into the process of getting to know each other. This can be a tricky one, regardless of whether it's heterosexual or homosexual.

Six months after being diagnosed with MS, Beth started dating a new man. There was a mutual attraction, but for Beth there were immediate questions: "What do I tell him and when?"

Beth and Matthew saw each other often for dinner and were becoming serious. They were in the midst of that full-disclosure process that is involved in every serious relationship. Who's the craziest family member? What are the family secrets? Who was the worst boyfriend or girlfriend? What are the worst emotional scars? Yet Beth remained unable to mention her MS. She attributed this reluctance to a fear of how Matthew might take the news, a desire to preserve her privacy, and to the fact that she had no idea how to tell the man she was dating.

A few weeks later, the issue came up during a visit with her MS specialist. He told Beth, "Well, you're never going to know until you tell him. Better now than later. If he's not up to the challenge, why get more involved?" Good question. Beth felt the same way. (This kind of common-sense help is another reason to find a specialist with whom you get along and whom you trust.)

Soon after the doctor's visit, Beth told Matthew about her diagnosis. In truly anticlimactic fashion, he accepted the news without hesitation, asked how he could help, and was upset only that she had not told him sooner. In fact, that was the only fight they had regarding the news. The last time I spoke to Beth, she and Matthew were still together.

IN A SENTENCE:

> By telling those in your immediate household now, you'll begin to get the compassionate support you need and reduce the stress of having a secret.

learning

Your Medical Team

NO ONE manages MS alone, as those who try to find out soon enough. So the sooner you begin to organize your support team, the easier it will be to cope with further tests, checkups, medication worries, insurance headaches, and mood swings.

MS is not the kind of condition where you can rely on just one health-care provider, either. Finding a good MS specialist is vital, but the medical team needs to be bigger. For example, what if your specialist is out of town when you need medical help or a prescription filled? The solution is another doctor or two, a nurse-practitioner, and even a friend with a medical background in your corner.

The sooner you have the medical team that works for you in place, the sooner the bumpy ride of these first few months with MS will smooth out. Let's look at the key members of your medical team.

Your MS expert

While there are many qualified neurologists, if you have MS, it is important to find a neurologist who *specializes* in the disease. Such a neurologist is involved with research into the disease and will be more current on possible causes of the disease and new treatments. Being in the care of an MS specialist who is aware of the latest studies of the origin and treatment of the disease will ensure you the best treatment available.

Your MS specialist will realize that your symptoms are serious and might lead to signs of MS. He or she will also be knowledgeable about how you feel about how MS has affected you. Obviously, this is helpful from a medical perspective. It is also key to your own personal comfort and peace of mind. Here is someone who knows. Here is someone who is familiar with what you are trying to explain. And here is someone you don't have to convince or try to make understand. He or she already is convinced and does understand. I cannot overstate the relief this can bring to the new patient.

My first meeting with the neurologist who became my MS specialist, Dr. Saud Sadiq, was such a revelation, even when he told me I had MS. I wasn't depressed—I actually found it exhilarating to hear him say, "You knew, and you knew you knew when the doctors didn't." I was relieved, because he knew, too. Finally, I had someone who could speak my language. I would no longer have to be translator as well as symptom sufferer and patient.

Finding an MS specialist is not as complicated as you might think. If you are lucky enough to have been diagnosed by a neurologist who specializes in MS, and you like him or her, stay with that doctor. Otherwise, ask your internist or the neurologist who diagnosed you for a recommendation. Local medical schools, other people with MS, and friends and family are other good sources for names.

Picking the right MS specialist is crucial in securing the best treatment. He or she will have a positive attitude that will help inspire a positive attitude in you. That's the positive partnership you deserve, and you should proceed with the attitude that you will settle for nothing less. Therefore, if you do not find a satisfactory level of trust and rapport with the first specialist you consult, get another recommendation and see someone else. Just as you wouldn't necessarily buy the first house you look at, you do not need to stay with the first specialist you see.

Your primary-care physician

Since continuity of care can result in better care, a good internist— a primary-care physician (PCP), in the language of managed care—is important for everyone, especially those with MS. If you're lucky, you already see someone you like and trust. The PCP is the linchpin of your medical team, the doctor you see most frequently for checkups and flus, infections, and other illnesses. If you're extremely fortunate, your PCP is associated with a variety of managed-care plans, so even if your insurance provider changes with a new job, you can continue to visit the same doctor.

Some of us are less lucky. As I described in the introduction, the internist I had when I fell down the stairs was disappointing, to say the least, during this big health crisis. I moved quickly to find someone new to be the linchpin of my medical team. My present internist is an excellent diagnostician. He is also a compassionate doctor who gives of his time and his medical expertise. He knows that you must treat the person as well as the disease, and that to do so you need to know your patient well.

It should be clear that having an internist you trust as a medical expert and as a person in whom you can confide is extremely important in your first year of living with MS. One reason to have a good PCP is that if and when you begin treatment with one of the **interferon-**based or other injectable medications, he or she will be the most readily available doctor to help monitor and treat side effects. For instance, my doctor saw me monthly after I began my treatment with Avonex (one of the now well-respected interferon-based treatments that can slow the progress of the disease). He always took blood during these exams to test whether my new medications were affecting other aspects of my overall health, such as liver function.

If you need to find a new internist, ask around for a referral. Ideally, you want a PCP who is experienced in dealing with patients who have chronic conditions. Friends, coworkers, family, and other health-care professionals may have someone to recommend. Your other doctors are the best source, and in fact it may also be easier at this point to confide in another physician that you now have MS, which will require special care.

Your gynecologist

Women need to have a gynecologist on their medical team and to see her or him for regular checkups. Since people with MS are particularly vulnerable to infections, this is important because a gynecologist is more likely to find such things as yeast infections and get you the proper treatment quickly.

It helps to have as much continuity in your life as possible. If you have been seeing a gynecologist for some time, someone whom you like and trust, he or she will be there for you as you navigate the brave new world after your diagnosis.

If you don't currently have a gynecologist, now is the time to find one. If your MS specialist works in an MS treatment center, the team of doctors there may well include a gynecologist who is a specialist in treating MS issues and symptoms particular to women. (This is true, for instance, at the Multiple Sclerosis Research and Treatment Center at St. Luke's–Roosevelt Hospital in New York City, where I am a patient.)

The National Multiple Sclerosis Society

THE NATIONAL MULTIPLE SCLEROSIS SOCIETY (NMSS) is dedicated to helping those living with MS to live healthier, richer, and happier lives, and part of that mission includes supporting new research into treatments for MS and, finally, finding a cure for MS.

If you join the NMSS, you will receive *MS Connection,* a very informative newsletter that offers a list of programs and services, including teleconferences and meetings on areas of interest as wide-ranging as "MS and Dating," "Horseback Riding," and "Managing Stress in the Workplace," as well as invitations to various activities sponsored by the NMSS. You will also receive the group's magazine, *Inside MS,* which offers a wide selection of helpful articles, interviews, book reviews on recent titles pertaining to MS, source guides for equipment, updates on research and treatment programs, and much, much more. NMSS will also send you periodic flyers inviting you to attend seminars on such varied topics as creative writing, furthering your education, and improving your work skills. The flyers will also inform you of various scholarships sponsored by the society.

Joining the NMSS is easy, and doing so will help you feel a real sense of accomplishment (however small it may seem at first!) in these first few days when you might feel you are just muddling through. Best of all, you can pursue getting the best MS care in your area. Call toll-free at 800–344–4867 (800-FIGHT-MS) or visit its website, www.nationalmssociety.org. Personally, I wish I had put aside my (unfounded) fears about being "typecast" and had joined sooner. By joining the NMSS, I've made friends, helped others–and been helped by them–and learned a lot!

Your psychologist or psychiatrist

Many people who are newly diagnosed with MS have found comfort in putting a therapist—a psychiatrist, psychologist, or other mental-health professional—on their medical-support team. Keep in mind that you have a lot on your plate right now and a period of depression following the diagnosis is not unusual.

For some, the depression may linger and begin to impair function, as well as diminish both any sense of well-being and the overall quality of life. Talking to a therapist can help you work through your anger, your fear, your mood swings, and any sense of despair that you might now be feeling. If you have any reservations about going to see a "shrink," it is nothing to be ashamed of—you need new kinds of support as you adjust to your diagnosis.

If it is warranted, your psychiatrist may prescribe a mild antidepressant or an anti-anxiety drug; other kinds of therapists may refer you to a psychiatrist who will prescribe the medication.

Clonazepam, an anti-anxiety medication, is one medication that both moderates anxiety and combats spasticity, a common symptom for those with MS.

IN A SENTENCE:

Assembling a medical team that you have confidence in will ensure a better treatment program and make you feel more secure.

Why Me?

WHEN YOU are newly diagnosed with MS, you may say to yourself, "Why me?" And you may hear yourself answer, "Well, why not?" Coming to terms with why all this happened will take time—more time for some people, less time for others.

After my diagnosis, my friend Felicia was great when I shared what I was going through with her. She held me when I cried, made me laugh, and took me out to more than one lunch. Her greatest gift was when she pointed out, "You didn't die in a plane crash. So, you're not dead yet, and you look great." The moment she said those words, I knew it was time to snap out of it.

The sooner you stop spending time wondering "Why me?" the sooner you will be able to use your energy to get yourself the best treatment possible.

The role of fate

When I was very young, my father had a friend who was a very wealthy entrepreneur. On vacation in the Swiss Alps, he was skiing alone when, evidently, he tumbled headfirst into a very deep snowdrift and suffocated to death in the snow—not even a broken bone, my dad said. I asked how this could have happened. My dad said, "Fate." I remember saying, "Fate must be very big." My dad laughed. I don't remember if I felt hurt or not, I think it was one of those nice dad laughs, but then I wondered why he had laughed. Now, I don't. I was right, the way a kid can be right, completely innocent of the import of a simple statement. Now, I understand, the joke is, there is no joke. It's true. Fate *is* big.

Many of us who had suspected all along that there was something serious going on or who have lived with a misdiagnosis such as Lyme disease, experience relief and cope with the "Why me?" part of the diagnosis very quickly, since we are anxious to get on with the treatment we've needed all along. This was the case for Bill. He spent six years with a diagnosis of Lyme disease. At first, he was asymptomatic, but as the years wore on, he began to experience symptoms that did not make sense. "I said to myself, if this is Lyme disease, I must have the worst case on record. I was having serious trouble walking and suffering fatigue. Heat always made me feel exhausted. I finally went to a neurologist in Boston and had a couple of spinal taps, and an MRI that got me a diagnosis of MS right away. I was pissed off that I'd wasted all that time when I could have been getting treatment, but since I'd known something was wrong all along, I didn't spend much time bemoaning my fate. I got started on Avonex right away. All I'm trying to do now is treat the goddamn disease." Since Bill had significant symptoms, including real trouble walking, his no-nonsense attitude was basically his only constructive choice. Being somewhat unique in that he was not diagnosed until he was in his late fifties, he didn't have the time or energy to feel sorry for himself if he wanted to keep walking, and he did.

This was not the case for Debra, who was only in her late twenties when diagnosed and who stated flatly, "I just still don't believe I have it." Though she had already had problems with her balance and her eyesight and had had an MRI that had shown the tiny white patches that characterize demyelination, she wasn't prepared to accept her condition. "I don't deserve this. This isn't me. I don't even want to talk about it." There wasn't much more to be said.

Charlie took a "let's just make the best of this" attitude, which was quite impressive, given what he had to face. Sadly, Charlie was diagnosed with MS when he was only twenty-one, but after a brief bout with melancholy, he said, "F— all this sadness." Charlie credits his mother a lot for helping him overcome the MS blues, actively pursuing treatment with disease-modifying drugs (he takes Copaxone), and embracing his ambition to be an actor. After a year spent stabilizing his condition at home in Michigan, he moved to New York. As he puts it, "I decided to take the big plunge, and my mom supported me every step of the way." When I met Charlie, he was working hard at a great job with the city's park services department and acting intermittently in off- and off-off-Broadway plays. "It's not easy, but then life never is," he said. Although he's had relapses and his acting career hasn't quite taken off, he remains undaunted. When he does have bouts with the blues, a talk and a good meal are all it takes for him to get his enthusiasm back. I admire Charlie. His path is not an easy one, either medically or professionally, but he stays on it and doesn't give up. He's a constant reminder to me that your attitude really can help.

Sydney also met her diagnosis head-on. Diagnosed in her midthirties, her "Why me?" answer was to try to find out. "Because I'm a research assistant to a history professor, I did what I always do. I did research. I am a white North American woman, fair skinned, of northern European ancestry, so all of that fits, but it doesn't explain why me and not, say, my best childhood friend who fits the same profile and grew up in the same town as I did. That's just fate." She gave a resigned, but wry laugh, which I shared.

I suppose my own answer to the question none of us can answer is similar to Sydney's, though, having been diagnosed in my forties, I share some of Bill's necessary resignation. Then there's the obvious fact that I have written a book about MS, certainly one way of facing the questions regarding the disease squarely, including "Why me?"

I also kept a file and I still keep one of accidents, illnesses, events in my past that might be clues to the larger why. In other words, viral infection is suspected of playing a role, particularly if it occurs in your adolescent years, and I had a terribly severe case of mononucleosis during my parents' difficult divorce. Mono is connected to the Epstein-Barr virus, which has been linked to MS in one Harvard study, but the linkage has not been proved conclusively. If there is a relationship to physical trauma, I was thrown from a horse when I was ten and suffered a minor concussion. The file is filled with countless entries of this nature and others that document periods of extreme stress that may have contributed to exacerbating my symptoms. Do I think I'm going to become the Sherlock Holmes who puts the clues all together and solves the mystery of MS? Of course not. However, we all owe it to each other to share with our doctors any unusual information regarding our personal history that might help further research into cause and cure in its own small way.

But the file does one important thing. When my doubts or my self-pity come to call, it gives me a simple way to find a place to lay to rest what otherwise might become obsessive musings.

When it comes to debating the "why did this happen to me" issue, perhaps an often quoted cliché says it best: "Don't question. Accept." When you can live with this, do. When you can't, go ahead and question. We all do, but we all must know that there are no real answers. Coping works a whole lot better than continually questioning fate.

How alone is alone?

You will find that these first days and weeks will leave you buffeted by a range of emotions and reactions. While, on the one hand, those who love you, as well as your medical team, will rally to you, there will be times when you are quite sure you are bearing this ordeal alone.

In those first few days I wrote in my journal a note stating that I felt I was incognito, feeling sick, shouldering a diagnosis, but living in the disguise of a well person. Here's an entry that describes this dual identity.

"I lead a double life. I'm ill, but no one can see that I am ill. There is no sympathy. Worse, there is no comprehension, no understanding. We all live our lives alone, but I am now alone within alone."

Keeping a Journal

MANY PEOPLE with MS keep a journal or diary. It's a convenient way to jot down physical symptoms and anything else you want to discuss with your doctor at your next visit. More important, a journal is a great outlet for you to deal with, and reflect on, your feelings about the disease and your life in general. Writing about your emotional state helps you process your feelings. In addition, it's often instructive later on, when in a particular mood or faced with a certain kind of situation, to reread your journal entries to see how you coped with similar things before.

You don't have to buy a special diary to keep a journal. A file on your computer will work just as well as a special notebook.

I assure you this has changed for good, and I share this only for comfort. You are not alone in feeling alone. It is a perfectly natural moment in your process of acceptance. Sometimes, this sensation will go away simply when you tell a friend "I feel so alone," and are reassured that you are supported by all who love you. Sometimes the feeling is more pervasive, particularly when you find confirmation of your "double life" status in how colleagues at work and others expect the exact same behaviors from you and that the demands made upon you will be met in the same old way. If the acceptance of your non-ill image leaves you feeling more and more isolated, you might want to consider consulting a therapist or finding an MS support group for the newly diagnosed, which you can find online or inquire about through your specialist's office.

The challenge

To help you move past the "Why me?" issue, you have to start thinking of what you are facing as a challenge. You still will experience moments contemplating this question, but being resolute can help you move beyond the question of why you were chosen to cope with MS.

In any event, there is no answer to the question of "Why me?" that any expert can give you, even now. The best thing then is to get on with the challenge.

IN A SENTENCE:

> At this point, no one can tell you exactly why you got MS, so the best thing to do is move on to treating it well and living well.

learning

Who Gets MS?

ENOUGH DATA is available that doctors and medical researchers have been able to reach some very tentative conclusions about when people usually become symptomatic and what kinds of people are more likely to contract MS. However, at this point, they do not know why MS strikes the people it does.

People generally develop MS between the ages of twenty and fifty. While the disease may be acquired as early as the teenage years, most of us become symptomatic only in our twenties, thirties, or even as late as our forties, fifties, and sixties. Often, people report certain symptoms to the doctor in their thirties, but are given a clean bill of health or a misdiagnosis; they end up living with MS without knowing it for a number of years.

There are several other factors that can predict the likelihood of contracting MS.

Gender

In some geographic areas women are twice as likely to be diagnosed with MS as men; in other places, women are three times more likely to contract the disease. It's not yet known why women are affected by MS so much more often than men, though hormones may play a part. Generally, women are more likely to be affected by all autoimmune diseases.

What the statistics do tell us is that men diagnosed with MS are actually more often diagnosed with the more severe forms of the disease, such as chronic-progressive MS. Men also tend to be diagnosed at an older age than women.

Women are more likely to be diagnosed during the childbearing years, the time of life when the hormones are constantly active. Often a woman may be diagnosed after a pregnancy and successful delivery. It is thought that the volatility of postpartum hormonal activity may activate the immune system and, therefore, trigger an episode that indicates MS. In fact, hormonal activity at menarche (the onset of menstruation), post-pregnancy, and pre-menopause may be related to the diagnosis of MS because of the intricate relationship between hormonal activity and the activation of the immune system.

Teenagers and MS

For years, multiple sclerosis has been considered an "adult disease," usually diagnosed in people between the ages of twenty and fifty. But with the advent of the MRI test and now even more advanced MRI techniques, the number of younger people diagnosed has increased somewhat dramatically. Now the National Multiple Sclerosis Society estimates that at least 8,000 to 10,000 teenagers in the United States between the ages of thirteen and seventeen have been diagnosed with MS; an additional 10,000 to 15,000 have MS, but have not been diagnosed.

At first reading, this is startling and disturbing, but the good news is that treatment at the very early stages of MS is most effective. Thus, it's better to know and get treatment. Here is one example: the professional race car driver Kelly "Girl" Sutton was diagnosed with MS at sixteen. Now, at thirty-four, she is in her third season of racing with NASCAR and is one of the few elite women racers. She also spends time talking with groups of young people with MS and has helped many kids motivate themselves to cope with their diagnosis and to thrive. So there, MS!

The NMSS publishes *Teens Inside MS,* a great magazine specifically for teenagers (see Resouces, page 246).

Missed Symptoms

WITH THE profusion of tests now available for ever more sophisticated neurological examinations, the number of people living in a limbo of "I know something's wrong, but I don't know what it is" is dwindling. Previously, a person might have experienced numbness, tingling, dizziness, or sudden vision loss, but because these symptoms would pass quickly, he or she would be given a clean bill of health. Luckily, things have changed.

The socioeconomic issue

The developed countries with high standards of living have the highest incidence of MS; poorer nations have a much lower incidence.

Once again, there is no clear answer about why this is so, only a few theories that remain to be researched and tested. Are residents of underdeveloped countries so poverty-stricken and subject to day-to-day illnesses that their immune systems haven't the time or the luxury, so to speak, to rebel against the body in the way that induces MS? Or is it that in areas with no running water or plumbing systems, people somehow develop an immunity to MS? Nobody knows.

Heart disease and diabetes are also more frequent in developed societies, but in those cases studies have suggested that the cause may be the high-calorie and high-fat diet prevalent in the West. More research needs to be done to determine the interplay between rates of MS and socioeconomic status.

Geography

On a similar note, it appears a person's chance of developing MS may have a connection to where one grows up. Residents of temperate climates, such as those of North America, Europe, and South Africa, are more likely to develop the disease than those in tropical climates, such as the equatorial zones of South America and Africa.

Even those people who spent their childhoods in tropical climates and moved to temperate areas later in life have a lower incidence.

One theory suggests that geographic location comes into play with people who already have a genetic vulnerability to the disease (for example, a first-degree relative with MS).

Within the United States, populations in northern areas are more susceptible than those living closer to the tropics. The 37th parallel, which runs from Newport News, Virginia, to Santa Cruz, California, seems to be a dividing line, with rates of MS higher to the north of this latitude than to the south.

Nevertheless, until such time as researchers determine why there seems to be this correlation between temperate locations and the prevalence of MS, it does little good for any of us to second-guess the place where we were born and raised.

Genetics

No gene directly linked to the development of MS has yet been identified. However, there may be genetic factors that affect one's risk of getting MS.

People with a first-degree relative (a parent or sibling) with MS have a *slightly* higher chance of contracting the condition. The risk is even smaller when a second-degree relative (grandparent, aunt, uncle, nephew, niece) has the disease.

Ethnicity

In the United States, whites are more likely to develop MS than people of color. African-Americans are half as likely to develop MS as are whites, and the incidence of MS in Americans of Chinese or Japanese descent is even lower—the rate of diagnosis is estimated to be one tenth that of whites. While few studies have been done to corroborate the following, it is estimated that Native Americans also have a low risk of getting MS.

The pattern for African-Americans is echoed in Great Britain, where blacks have a much lower risk of developing MS than whites. Interestingly, however, African-Americans do have a higher rate than blacks in Africa, which may point to geographic or socioeconomic factors.

Among American whites, those of Scandinavian origin seem to be particularly at risk. MS also does appear more frequently in Scandinavia. This does not mean that MS is your destiny if you are Scandinavian; my son's father is a Norwegian from Wisconsin, and no one in his entire extended family has ever been diagnosed with MS.

Other ethnic groups, such as Indians and Pakistanis, are at much lower risk. And there are populations that miraculously do not ever contract MS, including Eskimos, Gypsies, the Yakuts of Siberia, and the Bantus of southern Africa.

IN A SENTENCE:

> *Certain populations are at slightly higher risk of contracting MS than others, but as with so many other things about the condition, researchers don't know why.*

Telling Your Parents and Others

YOU'VE HAD a few days to adjust to your news, and you've told the people in your immediate family. Now is the time to tell your parents, your other loved ones, and anyone else in your personal life who may need to know soon, or with whom you want to share this new aspect of your life.

Your parents

Shalaylah told her parents in as straightforward a manner as possible. "My mother is a very excitable person, and I wanted to keep this as simple as possible. I was visiting them for the day. I waited until dinner was over, and I said, 'Mom, Dad, I have multiple sclerosis.' There was this sort of family squirm thing, and I added, 'But look how well I am. I'm doing well. I have great doctors. My insurance covers the medicine. I want you to know I'm going to be okay.' It took about a minute for my mom to wind up. 'Oh no. My god, that will leave you crippled.' I had to stop her. I told her, gently I hope, that that was not the case."

She tried to calm her mother down before she left. "I was exhausted after that." Then she sent her parents material to read about the disease-modifying medication she was taking. Her mother was less upset once she realized that there was real hope for Shalaylah to lead a healthy, normal life. "Sometimes I wonder whether I should have waited longer to tell them, but then I think, hey, I would have had to deal with it someday." Shalaylah's great advice on the subject of telling your loved ones: "Before you tell anyone, prepare yourself for any and every reaction."

Parents and children always affect one another's lives, throughout the individuals' entire life span. The emotional bond between your parents and you usually remains a strong one, even after you've grown up, started your own life, and settled into a career, family, or both. Your parents continue to see you as their child, a person whom they have to protect in this world, no matter what. Most parents have a love for their children so strong that it sometimes obscures a sense of limits and boundaries, even when those children left home long ago. This can complicate how parents deal with your diagnosis during this first year.

If you are in your twenties or early thirties, you may have recently landed the job you wanted, moved into the first apartment you could afford all on your own, or even just gotten married. You achieved independence and autonomy from your parents, but your diagnosis with MS has the potential to change things completely. You could find that your parents are suddenly back in your life in a big way—giving advice, telegraphing their worry, misplacing their concern, and perhaps subconsciously wanting you back in the fold. In short, you may be in the unenviable position of having to repeat your quest for adult independence.

The best way to maintain your status as an autonomous adult, while still being a loving daughter or son, is to show you are independent by example. If you are having a "bad" day, rely on your friends or your partner for emotional needs and support rather than calling home. Visit or telephone your parents on a "good" day, when you are feeling well and your positive attitude is happily intact.

People who are diagnosed in their late thirties or forties often face a different set of issues with parents. Your parents are older, so you may find yourself caught in the middle: your children are young and need a lot of attention, and your parents are developing chronic conditions as they age and may even require your help already. When you add in your own diagnosis, this can be a recipe for overload and stress. It's not easy to cope with all this at once, but it is possible.

Regardless of how old you are and what your parents' health status is, there are three common responses that parents of someone newly diagnosed with MS have.

1. *To become overbearing.* With an overbearing parent, a good thing for you to do is to cool it, but without being too obvious about it. Try to send a note or postcard, rather than calling as much as you might have before. Set limits when and how you can. If you have a sibling you love and trust, ask her or him to intervene. A sympathetic sibling can both run interference and talk to the parent(s) in a non-threatening way about what is and is not helpful to you right now. If you can talk about it with your parents, stress that MS is not going to kill you—you are going to cope, and cope well. In any event, keep in mind that their responses are the result of real love and of concern for your well-being—this may help you to be more patient with them.

2. *To panic about their own future.* Elderly parents or those who have already relied on you during major illnesses often panic when a child is diagnosed with MS. If one or both of your parents are already dependent upon you, offer reassurance that you're not going to keel over anytime soon. If they persist in their fears, give them pamphlets to read about MS, or take them to see your MS specialist for a discussion of your condition. Stress that you can still continue caring for them. Meanwhile, start getting help from others to protect yourself from being overwhelmed by the double duty of maintaining your own health and theirs, or make the time to research how you can do that in the future.

3. *To enter into a process of denial.* If your parents simply cannot or do not want to deal with your diagnosis, it may be a temporary relief to you (it's one less thing to deal with for now, as long as you can cope with the sense that they do not understand what you are going through) or a source of irritation. In the meantime, you have the freedom to make the adjustments you want to make to maintain your level of health and your healthy relationships, without any parental interference. But don't forget that eventually your parents will get past their denial.

Sometimes parental relationships may surprise you. If one or both of your parents offer helpful support, take it. Accepting your parents' desire to help may help you and it will definitely help them.

Telling the rest of the family

Before you tell your parents you have MS, there's one more thing to consider. Think about how, and from whom, you want others in your family to hear the news. You may want to tell all your relatives yourself, over a period of time. You may want your parent to tell your siblings, aunts, or uncles, so that you don't have to do so (these conversations can be draining). Or you may want to keep it a secret for a while, until the dust settles and you and your immediate family have had time to adjust.

Keep in mind that, upon learning that you have MS, your parents may naturally want to discuss the news with other members of the family. If you do not want your sisters, brothers, or other close relatives to know just yet, you have the right to ask that your mother or father keep it a secret.

On the other hand, parents often want to help. If you feel your parents can accurately convey the information and if you are feeling overburdened, you can ask them to tell other relatives. These people will probably call you directly, nevertheless, to convey their sympathy, ask more questions, and offer assistance; they may also give you a hard time for not telling them yourself (this is the downside of delegating the task to your parents).

This entire discussion on telling your family is based on the assumption that your parents, siblings, and other relatives *are* loved ones. However, if you are estranged from some of your relatives, be careful whom you tell, and only give the minimum information. You don't need any more hurt.

Telling friends

The first days after the diagnosis will leave you somewhat drained, in shock, and light-headed. It's important not to rush into anything, and this first week your goal is to choose not to decide anything you don't want to decide. You are in a waiting game you did not ask for or arrange. You are at the mercy of tests, reports, and doctors' findings. What you need from friends and family right now is simple: unconditional comfort and love.

In that light, choose wisely among your friends for whom to tell first and quickly. You will do well to have one, two, or three close compadres with whom you've shared other rough times, to whom you can speak in emotional shorthand, or with whom you can sit in a protective, peaceful silence. As a hippie friend with breast cancer said to me, "I know. Take the love. Love the love."

Other important people to tell

All your other doctors need to know about any preexisting conditions, so that they are aware of your complete health profile. (Your internist will probably have been the first to suspect there was something neurologically wrong and will not be surprised by your diagnosis.) You should also tell your dentist and discuss all dental procedures with your MS specialist ahead of time, in case there are precautions the dentist needs to follow.

You also need to tell anyone who works on your body that you have MS. It may sound paradoxical to be telling someone who gives you a shave or a manicure, but doing this will help you protect your health. For example, a manicurist should be even more careful not to nick you and break the skin, because this could put you at risk for infection, and infections can exacerbate your MS by triggering your immune system to go into action.

In addition to helping to prevent injury or infection, you need to make all of those who take care of you aware if you have special needs. For example, if heat triggers fatigue for you, you may want to suggest that the person who cuts your hair use a low heat setting when drying your hair or you may decide to leave your hair wet. You'll also want to suggest tepid water to soak your hands or feet in when having a manicure or pedicure.

IN A SENTENCE:

> *While you need to tell those closest to you, you should take your time doing so and be prepared for a number of varying reactions.*

learning

Diet, Exercise, MS, and You—A Preview

IT IS the fifth day since your diagnosis. While you recognize that you want to stay well and do what you can to retard the progress of the disease, it's not a good time to make enormous changes in your lifestyle. Still, eating right and staying fit are going to become increasingly important to you. What follows are some easy ways to eat better and get more exercise. These modifications are simple enough for you to introduce them into your daily routine right now. Later in the book, we will discuss diet (see Month 3 Learning) and exercise (Month 4 Learning) in more detail.

Upgrading your diet

These days it can be very difficult to choose the best things to eat. For years, you've been told that something is good for you, and then a new study comes out suggesting that the same foodstuff contributes to cancer or heart disease.

For now, try to ignore these controversies, since paying attention to all the nutritional debates can increase your stress levels. Instead, concentrate on making a few broad modifications in your diet, in areas where doctors, nutritionists, and the scientific community generally agree.

First, change the kinds of fats you're eating. Fat is a necessary part of the human diet, but there are good fats and bad fats. Reduce your intake of saturated fats, which are found in such foods as French fries and the fattier cuts of red meat. Fast food and junk foods are also full of saturated fats, which aren't good for anybody. In addition, some research shows that those with MS may have more difficulty digesting saturated fats than the rest of the population.

At the same time, increase the good fats in your diet: polyunsaturated and unsaturated fats. A good way to do this is to eat more fish, such as salmon, tuna, and trout. Walnuts, almonds, and Brazil nuts are other excellent sources of the better variety of fats.

It's through these foods that contain the "good fats" that you can obtain the omega-3 and omega-6 fatty acids. Make provisions to include foods that contain omega-6 fatty acids, such as leafy vegetables and whole-grain breads, in your diet.Don't overlook the even more important significance of omega-3 fatty acids. If you include flaxseed oil or capsules in your diet, you will be sure to get your omega-3s. Ocean fish also provide plenty of omega-3.

In general, most recent data suggests that when you are living with MS, it is helpful to limit your intake of saturated fat, particularly those from animal sources, and increase your intake of polyunsaturated fatty acids.

All the diets recommended for MS stress the importance of protein in the maintenance of healthy tissues and cell production. The problem with protein is it may come in high-fat or low-fat foods. Cut down on red meat and concentrate on low-fat sources such as fish, skinless white-meat chicken, and nuts. Switch to skim milk and other lower-fat dairy products, or else minimize your intake of high-fat dairy products.

Make fresh fruits and vegetables a dietary mainstay. Strike canned fruits and vegetables from your pantry. Use fresh produce, which has a higher nutritional value, whenever possible. If need be, "fresh frozen" is a reasonable compromise. When fixing meals at home, do not overcook vegetables, since doing so causes nutrient loss. Steaming is your best bet—and it's how you should ask for your veggies when you're dining out.

Include more fiber in your diet. Fiber is essential for a healthy digestive tract and, therefore, all the more important if you are managing MS. Fresh fruits and vegetables, legumes, lentils, and nuts are all fiber-rich foods. If you feel you are not getting enough fiber, you might try a psyllium-based fiber supplement, available at health-food stores and drugstores.

Finally, drink noncaffeinated liquids. Try to drink six to eight glasses of liquid a day as a digestive aid and for overall good health.

Exercise

If you want to manage MS well, exercise and staying active are vital to improving and maintaining stamina, endurance, flexibility, strength, and balance. It's much harder for disability to hit a moving target than a sedentary one. The stronger your limbs and body as a whole, the better you will be able to compensate for minor bouts with common symptoms.

If you've never exercised before, begin very slowly and you'll gain confidence. You can start by walking, for example. If your condition has already progressed, ask your MS specialist for recommendations on what you can do to maintain and even increase your physical strength.

If you were already exercising, try to do a little more. Think of your daily exercise routine as if you were training for a marathon—only in this case, your marathon is not a long road race, but the successful lifelong management of MS.

There's No Excuse Not to Exercise!

IN A recent article in *MS Connection*, the newsletter of the National Multiple Sclerosis Society, Stephen Kanter makes the point that while exercise at the gym, with a trainer, or with a physical therapist is of great importance, having exercise routines that you can do at home on your own is another invaluable component of overall fitness.

Ultimately, you are the one who has control over your exercise regimen. If you don't do it, nobody else can. Thus, it is extremely important that you make daily exercise a part of your life and keep it that way, no matter what your level of disability. For more information about exercising at home, go to www.athcare.com.

Whatever your previous level of physical activity, check with your specialist and your internist before starting any new exercise program.

Also, you'll want to put safety first. Use the proper equipment, including the right shoe or sneaker and well-maintained exercise machines. Make sure you exercise on a safe surface, one with give so that you will not injure muscles or joints. Don't exercise in excessive heat or cold. Finally, if you have heart palpitations, pain in a muscle or joint, or feel fatigued, stop exercising and rest. If palpitations or muscle pain persist, consult your doctor.

In the morning, before you even get out of bed, start your day with a series of stretching exercises and one or two simple yoga poses for balance and flexibility. You might begin simply by lying there and stretching your arms overhead, one at a time, and then bringing them back to the bed. Then, do the same for your legs by stretching, extending, and lifting the legs one at a time to a comfortable height and then returning the leg to the bed. Then flex the fingers and rotate the hands inward and then outward five times, or whatever is comfortable for you. Do the same with your feet. When you rise from bed, reach high and bend low, and do it again.

Options to consider immediately in terms of exercise include increasing the amount of walking you do in your daily life. Make sure you have the proper footwear to begin walking and protect against injury.

If you have access to a pool, go swimming. Swimming is an excellent exercise for those with MS, as it exercises the whole body, without putting stress on the legs or back, often areas of the body most affected by symptoms of MS.

You may also want to consider using a set of light free weights to pursue a weight-lifting routine to improve muscle strength. There are videos available that will help train you in an introductory free-weight routine that will get you started and keep you from injuring yourself. Working on a strength and flexibility routine that includes free weights to strengthen the lower body will be particularly important for you your whole life long.

Incorporate simple leg lifts into your exercise routine. Simply stand, holding the back of a chair if you need help with balance, and lift one leg until the knee and thigh are parallel to the floor, or as high as you can; then lower the leg. Repeat five times for each leg. This exercise helps keep your hip joints healthy, which is important for those of us with MS.

IN A SENTENCE:

> *Making simple changes in your diet and increasing your level of physical activity now will create a strong foundation for you to fight MS in the years to come.*

DAY **6**

living

Telling Your Employer and Business Colleagues

WHAT AND when you tell your boss and the people you work with every day will depend on the work you do, the kind of people you work with, and your own individual prognosis. You are in no way legally responsible to tell your employer about your diagnosis or condition. And, clearly, you'll want to wait to even consider this part of the process of disclosure until you have emotionally adjusted to the news yourself.

There is a wide variance of opinion about the advisability of mentioning your MS at the workplace, especially if you have few symptoms. Most experts—including doctors, therapists, and career counselors—do not recommend disclosure in your work life. They reason, first and foremost, that MS is your own business, not your business's business.

Unfortunately, myths about MS persist in public opinion. For example, years ago, MS was dubbed a "crippler of young adults." While the fact is that 75 percent of people diagnosed with MS will remain able to walk their entire lives, outdated notions about disabilities run strong in the business world. This is a major factor behind the advice not to tell your boss or any of your coworkers. Even in subtle ways, the knowledge that you have a disability may affect the size of your raise, your access to new jobs and promotions, and your entire career (despite the protections of the federal Americans with Disabilities Act).

Therefore, whether you have a desk job, work on an assembly line, or do something very physical like construction or teaching dance, you may have legitimate, practical concerns regarding employment and disclosure.

The arguments for telling your employer, and perhaps even your coworkers, that you have MS are simple. The principal reason is that you will not have to keep your health status secret. You will be able to focus more clearly and peacefully on both your health and your work.

If you have to take time off for tests or doctors' visits or you are suffering from a **relapse** or **exacerbation** (periods when your symptoms are worse), you won't have to make up an explanation for your absence from work. And if your condition is such that accommodation will make you more productive at work—whether it's a more flexible schedule or a change in responsibilities to lessen stress—you can more easily negotiate that.

In addition, there is that adage that honesty is the best policy. Advocates for the disabled observe that we owe it to one another to show the world that living with MS can be a positive, productive process. We are the examples who will not only destroy the stereotypes but inspire others.

MS *and the workplace*

Before making a decision about disclosing your medical status at work, consider how many years you've been working and what your career goals are. In a national survey published by the U.S. Department of Health and Human Services, about 40 percent of people with MS left the workforce before retirement age. More men than women were affected. This could be because men are more often diagnosed with **primary-progressive MS**, which is a more disabling type than the **relapsing-remitting MS** that is commoner in women. Or it may have to do with the nature of the work involved, since men are more likely to work at occupations that involve physical labor.

Not only do the symptoms and relapses of symptoms associated with MS contribute to job changes and job loss, but psychological factors, such as lack of motivation and depression, can contribute to the inability to hold on to a job.

Nevertheless, the situation in the workplace for those with MS is rapidly improving. Due to the combination of improvements in disease-modifying treatments and treatment for the symptoms of MS and due to the increasing pressure on employers not to discriminate against the disabled, it is more and more likely that a person with MS can remain in the workforce for as long as he or she wants.

Breaking the news

If and when you feel it is important to share your medical information at work, you'll want to try to take it step by step.

1. Talk to your doctor about possibilities in your treatment future that might necessitate your informing your employer. You don't want to spring a needed medical leave on an employer who has no prior knowledge.
2. Call your local MS society for a phone consultation to help assess the most constructive way of disclosing your condition in your individual case.
3. To test the lay of the land, confide in a friend on the job whom you trust. Not only should you gauge how your friend reacts, but ask for his or her opinion about how your supervisor may respond.
4. If your company has written policies about disabilities and medical leaves, review them. If you have questions, write them down for later. (In general, it's better to tell your immediate superior before discussing the matter with your company's personnel or human resources department.)
5. If the signs look good, make an appointment to see your employer. Rehearse what you intend to say—this is one situation where it is better not to say too much.
6. When the meeting comes, be as confident, calm, and businesslike as you can be. Focus on the positive: your commitment to your work; your absence of symptoms, or their minimal level; the prognosis for continued good health; and your confidence in your future as an employee. Focus only on symptoms that may affect your performance. Suggest positive solutions—for instance, if fatigue is your worst

problem, you might take a brief nap after lunch to stay productive in the afternoon, and add back the time at the end of the workday.

Inspiring examples

If you are contemplating divulging your MS status at work, you might want to read Michael J. Fox's *Lucky Man*. In this memoir, the popular actor recounts how he was diagnosed with Parkinson's early in life. He kept his news private for more than seven years, which is no easy feat for a public figure. Fox wanted to protect his privacy, and he was afraid of discrimination on the job.

His announcement generated a vast wave of support and sympathy. The star admits that going public with his illness has lessened the stress in his life and even given him a mission. He is committed to finding a cure for Parkinson's and to helping others with the disease. While his financial freedom is something few can identify with, the lifting of his burden of secrecy is something we can all understand.

The Actress Teri Garr provides more inspiration. After nineteen years of staying quiet for similar reasons, Garr announced in October 2002 that she had MS. In her recently published memoir, *Speedbumps,* with her trademark frankness and humor, Garr shares stories about being a working actress with MS, thus adding further insight on reasons you may not want to divulge your condition, and what to expect when you do tell.

IN A SENTENCE:

> *No one is better able to assess your work environment, and the proper way to share news of your MS there, than you are.*

learning

What Causes MS?

MS IS a fascinating illness, and the search for the cause and a cure has attracted some of the most brilliant medical minds of the last 125 years. To date, a definitive cause has not yet been established, but there is encouraging research going on. My own internist, Marc Siegel, told me, "Many experts feel that there is a constellation of causes that creates the onset of MS."

Getting diagnosed with a condition whose cause remains unknown to this day and that has no cure can be very frightening. But you can take comfort in knowing there are committed experts who will not rest until they've solved all the riddles of MS. And it can even be inspiring to join those dedicated researchers as they try to solve the mysteries of MS.

The causes of disease

All diseases are caused by something. Scientists have grouped the causes of human disease into eleven categories: allergy, congenital, degenerative, heredity, infection, metabolic, psychogenic, toxic, trauma, tumors, and vascular.

By now you probably don't need more evidence of MS's mysterious complexity, but consider this: every single category has been examined as a cause of the illness. The good news is that researchers have been able to eliminate most of these categories as the possible culprit behind MS.

While symptoms of MS may worsen and the symptoms in turn make a person's condition worse, MS does not begin via degeneration (Alzheimer's is an example of a degenerative disease). A person may have multiple lesions (demyelinated areas) and have no degeneration. Tumors, which may or may not be cancerous, are out, since with MS, it's the taking away of myelin rather than the growth of a foreign invader that begins to cause the damage. Although MS was investigated as a vascular disease (one involving the blood vessels), recent technological innovations (such as the MRI) ruled this out, and MS patients have been proven to have normal vascular systems. Nor are toxins the cause, because no theory involving toxic agents has withstood scientific investigation. (This does not rule out the possibility that some yet-to-be-discovered toxin plays a part in the development of MS.) While metabolic involvement was considered for a long time, it too has been rejected at this point.

Heredity has long been considered a leading possible cause of MS. However, as mentioned earlier, there is now evidence only of a slight increase in risk for the disease among first-degree relatives (parent, sibling). Even this added risk is probably environmental, since family members generally live in the same household and are therefore exposed to whatever mysterious component in that environment may be causing MS. There have been many studies, over a wide range of topics, of the effects of genetics vs. environment using identical twins. Generally twins have to share a condition 25 percent or more than other family members for a hereditary link to be determined. In MS studies, the numbers are nowhere near this percentage. Thus, despite continued suspicion of a genetic link, heredity has been ruled out as a possible cause of MS.

MS does not fit in with the profile for psychogenic disease (disease caused by an emotional condition) either—despite the fact that a person with MS may experience depression or increased stress. Congenital factors and trauma also seem highly unlikely. This leaves us with the possibility of an infection link or an allergic connection.

Genetic factors

It is probable that genetic factors play a role in increasing a person's chances for getting MS, but there is no specific marker and no single gene has yet been identified that might be responsible for the onset of MS. Thanks to advancing techniques, hundreds of genes can now be scanned in an effort to identify those genes that potentially contribute to the onset of MS.

Allergies

Allergies are responsible for a number of autoimmune diseases. As you have already learned in Day 1, autoimmunity is a medical situation where a body becomes allergic to its own healthy tissue; this causes the immune system to produce antibodies, which then proceed to attack this healthy tissue. Examples of autoimmune diseases are lupus, in which antibodies attack the small blood vessels, and rheumatoid arthritis, in which the joints are attacked by antibodies. In spite of strong evidence that MS is an autoimmune disease, no specific antibody for MS has yet been discovered.

Nonetheless, what is particularly intriguing to note is that some studies show that, prior to diagnosis, many people with MS are nearly impervious to allergy. This might be due to the fact that the immune system of people at risk for MS already works in odd, complicated, but as yet unknown ways. If this is true, it may be because our immune systems are strong—if anything, overactive rather than sluggish—that we develop MS.

Infections

The most probable cause of MS is considered to be an infection at an early age that remains dormant and, later on, causes an autoimmune response. According to this theory, the infection, which might be viral, starts the process and the autoimmune response perpetuates the condition.

It has long been thought that something in the environment must trigger or at least contribute to the onset of MS, and much data has been compiled that leads to identifying this environmental factor as most likely a form of infection, such as a virus, most likely experienced during the childhood years. This does not mean MS manifests itself at the time of the infection. It may remain dormant for years.

THE VIRAL CONNECTION

While there is as yet no obvious, definable "trigger" for MS—whether viral, bacterial, or otherwise—infectious agents are considered the number one suspect that triggers the faulty autoimmune reaction in people who are genetically predisposed to MS. Much research has been done and more and more studies are being devoted to the connection between dormant viruses that live in our systems and the onset of MS and its symptoms. Some studies are under way that include an ongoing dose of an antibiotic as part of the overall treatment for MS.

Viral infection has risen to the top of the list of suspects as a result of the geographical distribution of the disease and the fact that clusters of multiple sclerosis were identified in the Faeroe Islands, the Danish archipelago between Scotland and Iceland, between 1943 and 1989. But by far the most interesting reason is that viruses are very similar to myelin—the protein that MS attacks. It is thought that a virus may cause the confusion in the immune system that characterizes MS so that the T cells of the immune system begin to attack their own myelin rather than the intruder virus.

The infectious agents under scrutiny are

The Epstein-Barr Virus (EBV). EBV is perhaps the most provocative virus under investigation. The majority of those diagnosed with MS display some evidence of EBV infection, which is also the cause of mononucleosis. At this time, further studies are exploring this possible connection.

Herpes Virus 6 (HHV-6). The cause of the benign condition of roseola in children, HHV-6 can also cause encephalitis (which involves brain inflammation) in patients with impaired immune systems—hence the possible connection. In addition, other herpes viruses—Herpes 1 and 2, as well as the varicella-zoster virus that causes chicken pox and shingles—may infect brain cells. There is still no hard evidence proving these connections, and experts are continuing to investigate.

Chlamydia Pneumoniae. While there are higher rates of the chlamydia infection in those diagnosed with MS, there is no hard evidence of any causal relationship. Still, because a chlamydia infection can cause ongoing inflammation, research continues.

There are other agents under investigation, but so far studies have been inconclusive regarding any connection with causing MS.

IN A SENTENCE:

Although the cause of MS remains unknown, research is focused on the possibility that viral or bacterial infections trigger the process, perhaps years in advance of the first appearance of symptoms.

Coping with Fear

FEAR CAN take many forms. Ignoring it is impossible, especially at this time of your life. But while fear is natural and inevitable right now, facing it and understanding it will mean that it won't overwhelm you.

In this first week of living with MS (and probably for the weeks to come as well), you will find that your fear will come in different sizes at different times and that it will visit you for myriad reasons. While what you fear and how much you fear is unique to you, there are certain issues involved in MS that cause all of us who are diagnosed to experience at least some level of fear and trepidation.

Types of fear

You have already experienced one type of fear, the one we all have when we are going through the battery of tests that the doctor assures us will help determine what the matter is. No one gets through a diagnosis of MS without a substantial dose of this fear of the unknown. My own fear put me in a sort of numb, detached state—I seemed to float above myself, watching myself move from appointment to appointment and listen to doctor after doctor. I was without moorings. My sense of personal identity was cast adrift.

Once I had my diagnosis, the fear of the unknown dissipated. Sure, there were still a lot of unknowns—what the disease was like, how it would affect me, etc.—but at least I could work to master my own fate. With my feet planted firmly on the ground once more, I was relieved and could plan for an active, positive future.

Another type of fear is the "Oh my god" kind, as in "Oh my god, I've got this dreadful disease." This one can be worked through by realizing that it's not dreadful—it just *is*, it's the way things are now. Your actual health status at the end of this week is the same as it was at the end of last week. It's just that now you have a label, a name for it. Remind yourself of this when you feel the "Oh my god"'s or "Oh no"'s coming on.

The fear of rejection or the fear of judgment affect many people who are newly diagnosed. They worry about how their loved ones and the people who populate their personal and professional world will react. We all have such fears at one time or another, but this is not the time to let them fester. You don't need or deserve the added burden. In fact, if anyone reacts oddly or unsympathetically to your news, he or she is the person with the problem—not you. (As mentioned earlier, a loved one who cannot adjust to your news should get help, whether from a member of the clergy or a therapist, or by seeing your MS specialist to learn more about the disease. Do not make this your problem. You have enough to manage.)

The biggest fear people with MS feel right after they learn the diagnosis is the fear of the future. We all question destiny, what the future holds, where we will be in terms of our life goals in the years to come, but now your situation is different. In addition to all the other ponderings over what is to come, a new one has been added—will I become disabled and what will my disability level be?

This is the kind of question that asks itself usually late at night when everyone else in the house is asleep, and your imagination is wide awake. Since even the experts can't predict the course of MS, it's best to brush this one off by saying, "Who knows? I'll simply do my best." If that doesn't work, get out of bed and write down your fears in your journal and then try to sleep.

This fear of the future will invariably return. It is best managed by remembering research on disease-modifying treatments has improved the overall health profile of those with MS. In addition, finding a cure for the disease is near. In the meantime, the newest treatment strategies work so well that they may be considered to be almost as good as a cure.

As long as you manage your general health and, once it's determined, the specific treatment of your MS, you are in the best position to trade the fear of the future for the worries everyone has: financing your children's college education, the usual problems of advancing age, and so on.

Surrendering your fear

We all know that control is an illusion, but it is an illusion most of us cherish. And that's okay, because sometimes it helps to maintain an emotional balance, if nothing else. Of all the emotions that fiddle with our sense of having some control, fear is perhaps the most prominent. There are situations that cause legitimate fear that are far worse than being diagnosed with MS, like the fear of war, natural disaster, or terrorist attack. But that doesn't mean your diagnosis isn't a justifiable reason to be fearful.

"What I'm most afraid of is not being able to walk," says Beth. Diagnosed at thirty, she has every reason to consider this possibility. "I think of the future, wondering whether I will ever get married, or not even get married, just find someone to love who'll love me back. Will I ever have children? How will my career change? What will people think when they find out? Will my friends' feelings toward me change? But it always comes back to, Will I be able to walk twenty years from now? Then my mood changes. I don't know . . . I rest. I feel better. Suddenly, I have a lot of energy, and that makes me feel triumphant, and I decide: Yes. I'm walking now, and I'll keep on walking."

Beth is one of us. Our fears may manifest themselves differently, they may come and go, but we have to recognize that they are there. If you've had an episode, you may fear a relapse. If you've taken a fall, you may be afraid of falling down again. You may wonder how your coordination will be affected. You may be afraid of how your condition may affect your career path. You may wonder about your sex life, your social life, whether you'll have to walk with a cane. If you are athletic, you may be afraid you won't be able to continue to remain as active as you want to be. You may dread the idea of needing a cane all the time. You may fear incontinence. You may fear pain. Your fears may run the gamut from embarrassing yourself in public by losing control of your bladder or taking an ugly fall to "Am I going to die from this?" Anything and everything may cross your mind, and this is normal.

You are not going to die. There are ways to manage bladder control and other symptoms. There are medications for pain, spasticity, and other problems you may face. Your life will probably go on much the same as usual, but you must also accept your fears and allow yourself the time to adjust to your new situation. You didn't get MS overnight, and you can't expect yourself to come to terms with having MS overnight either.

This is your period and process of recognition. Some therapists say you have to surrender to your fear first before you can let go of it. But if this sounds too trendy, think of it as meeting your fear on even ground. Ariel, another thirty-year-old who had recently been diagnosed, said, "Yes, I'm afraid sometimes, but that's okay, because my fear is not my boss." You don't have to hug your fear; just allow it residence, because believe me, the fear of those first few days or weeks is stressful. Don't be surprised if fear is a frequent visitor at your house right now. A visit is fine—just don't allow fear to be a permanent resident.

A *place in the world*

To quell your fears and begin to live comfortably and in harmony with your condition, remind yourself now and again that we all live in an uncertain world at best. You might even consider yourself ahead of the game in coping with uncertainty in general, since your condition puts you in a perfect position to deal constructively with a crazy world.

As you look at your fears and accept them for what they are and hopefully move beyond them, it's important to hold on to your sense of self. Perhaps Julie Full-Lopez put it best in her essay "Setting Goals": "In counseling, I was beginning to understand that I was letting fear of the unknown . . . change the way I saw myself, change the sense of my own identity." Don't let this happen to you. If you feel you are losing the battle with fear, do what Julie Full-Lopez did and seek help. (You can read the rest of her essay in editor Margot Russell's collection of essays by men and women with MS called *When the Road Turns*—see For Further Reading.)

IN A SENTENCE:

> *By managing your fears and putting your health situation in perspective, you will be better able to adapt to living with MS.*

learning

How to Relax

YOU'VE MADE it through a very difficult week, so first off you deserve a pat on the back. Take the time to congratulate yourself for having weathered the storm of diagnosis. Now is the time to catch your breath and gather your forces. The best way to do that is to relax.

As has been mentioned before, rest and relaxation will be an important part of your treatment plan. Taking a rest need no longer be seen as indulgent, and it is an absolute necessity for fighting stress and ensuring your good health when living with MS.

Learning to relax

Go soft focus, and don't addle yourself about tomorrow. By letting yourself relax today, even forgetting (to whatever extent you can) that you have MS, you'll rejuvenate yourself and feel stronger for the week ahead. So, sip a cup of tea and let go. There will be plenty of time to worry about things tomorrow, but for now, be yourself and relax.

Many of us have forgotten the simple virtue of relaxation. Think of your diagnosis as your opportunity to relearn what generations before us took for granted as part of a healthy life—the ability to enjoy simple, quiet moments while sitting with a friend, whittling, knitting, quilting, gardening, mending, or simply sitting still. Remember, relaxing is all about being idle without really being idle.

Need help doing so? Here are some tips:

○ If you have children, play with them. Spending time with a niece, nephew, or the child of a friend is also a great way to forget about your troubles.

○ Play with your pet. (If you don't have one but have wanted to buy or adopt, this may be the right time to do so.)

○ Read poetry. A poem can change your mood. A poem can give you intellectual food, a boost of mental energy. And a poem can take your mind off everything for a moment of utter concentration and contemplation. In a world suffering from a decreasing attention span, a poem that grips you and turns around how you think about something, if only for a minute, can actually increase your attention span.

○ Read P. G. Wodehouse, particularly the Bertie and Jeeves series. These books will take you far away from the reality you manage every day.

○ Go to the movies. Walk out if you don't like the film.

○ Watch a sporting event on TV.

○ Go to a museum.

○ Go to the zoo with family or friends.

○ Read a magazine you never have time to read.

○ Read a favorite cookbook.

○ Go through all those old catalogs you've been saving.

○ Surf the Internet, if you find that relaxing. (If you find it isolating, then pick a more social activity.)

○ Buy some Silly Putty and knead it when you're nervous or anxious. Not only will the simple motion help relax you, but this exercise also helps finger dexterity!

○ If you are able to, take a walk in a public garden or park.

○ Take up an old or new hobby. Knit, crochet, garden, anything that takes your mind off you.

○ Practice simple yoga poses.

○ Listen to your favorite music.

○ Light aromatherapy candles. Pick your favorite scent, whether or not it promotes "peacefulness." Just remember to blow them out before you leave the house or lie down for a rest.

○ Research those piano/guitar/harp lessons you always wanted to take.

○ Put all those photos into that photo album you bought, but never filled.

○ Have a "visit" on the phone with an old friend who lives far away.

There are many other ways to relax. Be imaginative. No matter how you choose to relax, bask in the moment.

Taking the day off

Michael told me that one day during that first grueling week, he threw his hands up in the air and went "Argh!" Then he decided to refuse to think about MS (or at least try) for an entire day. "I ordered out Chinese. I watched a bunch of movies on my new DVD player. I took the pill my doctor had given me for sleep before going to bed. It was great. I was glad I allowed myself to do that."

Try to follow Michael's lead and "take the day off." This doesn't mean you stop functioning and go lie down. It means you let go of your mind a little more. Even if it's a weekday and you've got work, school, or kids to deal with, carve out some time for yourself to let go and be yourself. For at least a few hours, be absolutely frivolous and play!

Here are some suggestions. Whatever you choose to do with your time off, be enthusiastic.

○ Start a book you never planned to read.

○ Rent a favorite movie or comedy collection and watch it during the day!

○ Take a walk for no reason with no real destination.

○ Bring your first cup of coffee or tea back to bed and sip it slowly.

○ Take a nap, if you feel like it, as long as it's early enough in the day not to interfere with your night's sleep.

○ If you're used to cooking, order out.

○ If you always order out, find a simple recipe and cook a simple meal at home.

○ Go out to dinner with your partner/lover, your children, your whole family, or a favorite friend.

After you've had your time off, hold on to the benefits of relaxing. Take a positive attitude to bed with you, and get a good night's sleep.

The power of laughter

It's amazing to me how many people seem to have forgotten to laugh or, even worse, seem to think laughing is beneath their status as a serious, thinking individual. In fact, laughter is the highest art and, as the old adage has it, "the best medicine."

Without laughter we would be at the endless mercy of our sorrows. In addition, it's good for your health.

So watch a silly movie, look at classic TV comedy series (anything you've enjoyed, from *The Honeymooners* to *Absolutely Fabulous*), watch the latest on the Comedy Central network (even if you don't think you like it), or invite a funny friend over for a visit. By embracing laughter, you'll relax and feel better.

IN A SENTENCE:

> *Making room in your life for time to relax and unwind is the best way to cope with the fatigue and stress of MS.*

FIRST-WEEK MILESTONE

By the end of your first week, you have begun to take control of your MS as you have now:

○ LEARNED THE BASICS OF WHAT MS IS AND ISN'T, AND UNDERSTOOD THAT THERE IS STILL MUCH MYSTERY SURROUNDING THE CONDITION.

○ BEGUN TO PUT TOGETHER A MEDICAL TEAM OF EXPERTS TO ENSURE THE BEST COURSE OF TREATMENT POSSIBLE.

○ LEARNED ABOUT WHY THERE ARE STILL TESTS TO UNDERGO AND WHAT THESE TESTS MAY ENTAIL.

○ ALLOWED YOURSELF TIME TO EXPERIENCE SHOCK AND DISBELIEF AT YOUR DIAGNOSIS. YOU DO NOT BLAME YOURSELF FOR YOUR ILLNESS.

○ TOLD THE PEOPLE WHO NEED TO KNOW IMMEDIATELY ABOUT YOUR CONDITION IN ORDER TO GET THE HELP YOU NEED.

○ FOUND WAYS TO ACCEPT AND LIVE WITH THE INSECURITY OF NOT KNOWING EXACTLY WHAT THE DISEASE YOU HAVE IS OR WHAT THE FUTURE HOLDS.

○ ACCEPTED FEAR AND LET GO OF IT SO THAT IT WILL NOT RULE YOUR LIFE.

Debunking MS Myths and Stereotypes

YOU KNOW a lot more about MS than you did a week ago, but you're well aware that much remains unknown about the condition. As your family and friends get used to the idea of your diagnosis, you will probably have to confront a number of myths and stereotypes about MS. All of us with MS function as public ambassadors for the disease, in that it's part of our "job" to educate everyone else. While this may seem like another unnecessary burden, it's more of an opportunity for you to get your family and friends on your team as emotional support. If you help them learn what is myth and what is true, they'll be in a better position to help you when you need it.

Even with casual acquaintances, you'll be breaking down myths and debunking stereotypes each time you answer someone's questions truthfully.

The cripple myth

"Oh my god—MS! That will cripple you."

If you haven't already heard these words, you soon will. Be calm, remembering that this reaction is because the person knows less about the course of the disease than you do, not because he or she is trying to hurt you.

Tell the person you don't walk with a cane right now, and that you probably won't even in twenty years. While it's possible you might eventually need a cane, there is a 75 percent chance you will never need a wheelchair and that you will remain walking your whole life.

Tearing down the cripple myth is a common task for those with MS. Each time you do so, you are not only combating ignorance but also working to ensure that fewer and fewer of us are discriminated against.

While we don't deserve to be discriminated against, it can happen as long as the cripple myth and its accompanying overtones of disability remain strong. Therefore, when you're in this situation, speak up with the facts, but don't yell. Carry on proudly, as your actions will speak louder than anyone else's words.

If you ever do feel discriminated against, keep in mind that awareness of the rights of the disabled is becoming a norm. The Americans with Disabilities Act gives us certain protections. We also have the tools and the medical support to keep disability to a minimum and, quite possibly, eliminate it from our future entirely.

The "moodiness" stereotype

You have probably reacted to your diagnosis with some combination of shock, fear, anger, dread, despair, and who knows what other emotions. It would be crazy not to do so when confronted with such news. Common sense makes it clear that you have to run the gamut of emotions to become comfortable with the new place you find yourself in.

By now your mood swings will once again be resembling those of any other person. Don't let anyone stereotype you as too emotional, or too moody. Everybody has moods and mood swings, and you are entitled to yours.

Louise, who was forty-one at the time she was diagnosed, found that whenever she expressed any frustration or anger, her husband or mother kept asking, "Are you angry at me because you have MS?" She reports that one day she finally told her mother "the truth: 'No, I'm angry at you because I'm angry at you.' It helped me feel free to be myself."

Louise's response is valid. The best thing to do in such situations is to accept that you are doing the best you can with what you have. You are entitled to have your emotions, but try to stay calm in dealing with those around you.

The "your personality brought this on you" stereotype

Perhaps the most pernicious stereotype regarding MS says that there is something ingrained in the character of people with MS that causes them to get the disease. While I was researching this book, I was appalled to read one author's claim that many people with MS have lived lives in which their dreams and ambitions have not been met or in which, they feel, despite all their Type A drive, they've yet to achieve what they meant to achieve.

This is complete hogwash. Bah humbug.

To make it clear that this is nonsense, take a look at some of the famous people who have come down with MS. Among entertainers, who could be more disparate in character and career than the late Richard Pryor and the former Mouseketeer Annette Funicello? They had in common that they achieved some reasonable worldly success, *not* that their personalities somehow induced the disease.

Take the writer Joan Didion and the late politician Barbara Jordan. Yes, both of these talented women have been advocates for causes right and just, but beyond that nothing in their personalities unites them.

Finally, take the talk-show host Montel Williams and the fictional President Josiah Bartlet in the old TV hit *The West Wing*. Not only is there the obvious difference that one person is real and the other fictional, but here too there is no common thread beyond the initials MS.

Don't allow yourself to believe that a certain type of person gets MS. There is no such thing as the MS type, and thank goodness for any blessings.

IN A SENTENCE:

> *The only thing you have is MS, but you may have to continually confront and defuse myths and stereotypes about the disease.*

learning

Your Treatment Options: Disease-Modifying Medications

UNLESS THE onset of your MS was particularly severe, you most likely will not start any treatment right away. How long the options are considered depends on the severity of your episodes and your symptoms. In most cases, it takes time to decide which drug is the best one for you. The most important thing to remember is that you have a say in the choice of treatment: it's your case, your illness, and your body. You want to gather as much knowledge as possible on treatment choices, from more than one source, but without overwhelming yourself. It's worth waiting a few weeks to try to get enough information to make the right choice for you.

Your MS specialist is the primary source for information on your medication options. In addition, you may read up on a specific drug, either in a drug reference book at your public library or on the Internet. And a concise review of the most widely used treatment options follows.

There are two major types of therapy for MS, symptomatic therapy and disease-modifying therapy.

Symptomatic therapy does just what it sounds like it does—treats the symptoms of MS. Symptomatic therapy, including the use of steroids, also known as cortosteroids, to relieve symptoms, is discussed in detail in Week 3 Learning.

Disease-modifying therapies actually work to change the course of the disease by slowing down its progress. Instead of treating the symptoms, the therapies treat the *cause* of the symptoms—the disease. In turn, these therapies can help to minimize the number and severity of exacerbations and therefore help control symptoms in that way. The two major therapies are interferon-based injections and glatiramer acetate (Copaxone).

Interferon-based treatments

In order to learn how your treatment may work, let's add to what you already know about the workings of the immune system. *Cytokines* are the immune system's hormones. They help regulate the responses of the immune system to inflammatory conditions and viruses.

Interferon is a kind of cytokine. The body produces this protein when it must react to a foreign agent, such as a virus, or a foreign substance. Beta interferon is said to "calm" the immune system, which is clearly a necessity in managing MS well. As a result, the interferons are called immunomodulatory agents: they "modulate" the immune responses.

Interferon-based treatments have been proven to substantially modify the course of the disease in many cases. There are three major kinds of interferon currently available for treating MS:

1. Avonex is the trade name for the beta-1a form of interferon. It is administered once a week, by **intramuscular deep (IMD) injection.** As simple as it sounds, one of the great advances in MS treatment is the way we can now administer our medicine. When I started out with Avonex in 2000 I had to mix the dose, tap the syringe, and then get down to the difficult and real business. Now Avonex is sent to you by your insurance company's affiliated pharmacy in pre-filled syringes.
2. Betaseron, the trade name for interferon beta-1b, was the first medication approved for treating MS with the two goals of minimizing symptoms and slowing the progress of the disease. Betaseron is

injected three times a week by **subcutaneous injection (SI)**. Its side effects, such as flulike symptoms, are easily manageable.

3. Rebif, another interferon beta-1a, is a newer drug approved by the Food and Drug Administration for use in the United States after studies showed promising results. Rebif has a short-term advantage over Avonex in reducing relapses, but after twenty-four weeks the drugs seem to work equally well. Rebif is taken three times a week by SI. As with Betaseron, redness and irritation at the site of injection may be an ongoing issue. You can now receive your Rebif in pre-filled syringes, which really do help make your life easier.

Glatiramer acetate

Marketed under the name Copaxone for treatment of relapsing-remitting MS, glatiramer acetate is a substitute antigen that mimics the proteins of the myelin sheath. By protecting myelin from demyelination, this treatment facilitates the fight against degenerative symptoms of MS. It serves to inhibit the immune reactions responsible for tissue damage and the production of additional plaque, which creates new lesions via demyelination.

While the interferons work by affecting the entire body's immune system, glatiramer acetate is thought to modify only those elements in the immune system's activity that are considered responsible for MS and its symptoms.

You can also receive your Copaxone in pre-filled syringes. Copaxone must be injected every day subcutaneously. The needle you use is a fine one, and the procedure is similar to that of injecting insulin for diabetes. The most common side effect is a brief redness and irritation at the injection site.

Tysabri (natalizumab)

The newest possible medication option for treatment of MS is Tysabri (previously called Antegren). Tysabri is generally recommended for patients whose response to other disease-modifying drugs has been insufficient or who have not been able to tolerate other disease-modifying treatments. Tysabri is a monoclonal antibody, not an interferon-based treatment. Monoclonal antibodies can be designed to bind with receptors on the body's normal cells and used to alter normal or abnormal cellular responses. Tysabri works at the cellular level to prevent leucocytes (immune cells) from migrating from the bloodstream to the brain, where the nerve damage that causes MS can occur. This is why there has been such excitement around the development of this drug. Tysabri is administered intravenously approximately every four weeks in your doctor's office.

However, it remains only a possibility for treatment. Tysabri was available in the United States for a short time in 2004, but was almost immediately withdrawn by the FDA after being linked in some patients to a rare and serious brain infection called progressive multifocal leukosencephalopathy (PML). Tysabri had been found to be effective for relapsing forms of MS (relapsing-remitting and secondary progressive) in reducing the occurrence of clinical relapses and in slowing the progression of disabilities connected with MS. However, after a small number of patients in the drug's clinical trials developed PML, the FDA withdrew the drug.

In early 2006 the FDA lifted its hold on new clinical trials of Tysabri; by the end of June 2006, the drug was approved for marketing in the European Union. As of this writing, clinical trials of Tysabri are continuing in the United States.

Notwithstanding the uncertain status of Tysabri, there is a program that makes the drug available for those for whom it might be the best medication option. Biogen Idec, Inc., the manufacturer of Tysabri, now sponsors a risk management program called the TOUCH Distribution Program, which offers restricted distribution of the drug. Developed in conjunction with the FDA, TOUCH allows doctors and their patients access to Tysabri while following stringent safety guidelines to ensure patient safety. Under the program, prescribers must be registered with TOUCH and must comply with a series of safety requirements; in addition, only infusion centers registered with the program can administer the drug. Safety surveillance includes systematic tracking of all patients taking the drug, and the monitoring and reporting of all occurrences of PML, as well as reporting any and all other infections. The goal of the program is to make Tysabri available to those who may benefit, while minimizing the risk of PML.

If you are having issues with your present medication, consult your specialist for further information on this program. But unless your doctor and you feel that Tysabri could result in a marked improvement in your condition, it's best to play it safe and wait until all the results are in and analyzed.

You can find out more on Tysabri by going to the NMSS website, www.nationalmssociety.org, and searching for Tysabri.

Good Intentions

BACK WHEN I was a tenderfoot on the MS trail, Rebif was the newest, hottest treatment about to become available for MS. Many well-meaning friends would send me articles on this new wonder drug or, even worse, bring articles to lunch dates to show me, so that I would have to face this serious material before I had even ordered my meal—a choice I find hard enough to make under the best of circumstances. When you've settled on a course of treatment with your trusted doctor and grown comfortable in your routine, the last thing you'll want is to be confronted with doing more research, asking more questions, and, worse still, perhaps doubting your trust in your chosen physician. Personally, my doctor and I are both happy with the results I am achieving with Avonex and as well intentioned as friends' advice may be, I do better when I don't second-guess my doctor or myself. Good results are good results.

It is important to remember that you are the one who is becoming the patient/expert, and that no one knows better than you and your doctor what the right course of treatment is for you. However, your doctor will definitely explore treatment options with you, including Tysabri, if appropriate and available. Until then, it's best to watch and wait. It's okay to simply say to concerned friends who advise specific courses of treatment, "Thanks. My doctor knows all about it" or "My doctor and I are on top of it."

Even more important, during your first year of coping with MS, your new routine, and all the information you have to absorb, a little knowledge—while not a dangerous thing—might just be depressing. The last thing you need is to scare yourself any more or have well-meaning friends do it for you. Remember, it's most important to stay on the positive side of the street right now.

Choosing which medication to use

The choice of what medication you take is up to you and your doctor. While your doctor cannot make you take a certain medication, his or her opinion is of great value—after all, it is your physician who has evaluated your case thoroughly. Chief among the factors to consider is what kind of injection you will be administering (subcutaneous or IMD), and how many times a week you will be injecting.

In certain cases, when the onset of MS is severe, you may be hospitalized until the situation is stabilized. Cortosteroids may be administered intravenously and Betaseron may be the medication of choice precisely because it is injected every other day. Once you are stabilized and discharged, your doctor may recommend a switch to Avonex as your long-term medication, because a dose of interferon beta-1a is no longer necessary every other day.

Don't forget that just because you start on one medication doesn't mean you can't change to another later in your treatment. In cases where side effects are severe, you and your doctor will reevaluate your situation and consider a different medication. (See Month 9 Learning, "Other Medication Options.")

This table may assist you in comparing your disease-modifying medication options.

Your Medication Options

BRAND	GENERIC NAME	MANUFACTURER	YEAR APPROVED	APPROX. COST PER YEAR
Avonex	Interferon beta-1a	Biogen	1996	$16,977
Betaseron	Interferon beta-1b	Berlex	1993	$32,388
Copaxone	Glatiramer acetate	Teva Pharmaceutical Industries	1996	$21,600
Rebif	Interferon beta-1a	Serono, Inc.	2002	$9,828
Tysabri	Natalizumab	Biogen	2007*	$28,392*

*Projected date and price, pending FDA approval

The injection

The idea that you will be responsible for injecting yourself with your own medication can be difficult to get used to. Keep in mind that incorporating self-injection into your treatment plan will make you more independent and self-sufficient.

A nurse in your specialist's office will train you in how to give yourself your injection, during one or two visits, or until you feel confident you can do it on your own.

It may be hard to fathom, but you will be safe injecting yourself and you will get used to it.

One patient's experience

Once my MS specialist explained the various treatment options, I read up on the medications and did some research on the Internet. Dr. Sadiq had recommended Avonex for me. I wound up going with his choice for two main reasons. First, I was diagnosed early with few symptoms, and Avonex was the only treatment option available that has been proven to slow the progression of disability. I also preferred to have one injection a week, rather than one daily or every other day.

Nevertheless, my first six months on Avonex were difficult. In order for my body to adjust to the medication, the first month I started out on a quarter dose, and then a half dose. But once I went on the full dose, I had the full range of side effects, led by (as I was warned) nausea.

I had picked Saturday afternoons as the best time to give myself my weekly injection, because that gave me all day Sunday to recuperate.

I took two tablets of Tylenol before the shot to avoid a severe headache afterward. Once I gave the shot, I lay down to rest (although I could rarely sleep). There was a headache, but it was controllable, and I also had chills and shivers. The problem ensued a few hours later, after a light dinner. First, a tad of queasiness. But then the big whammy of nausea, and I'd have to run to the bathroom to vomit.

Although this was no fun, I stuck with Avonex. For one thing, the day after the shot, I was okay. For another my doctor was quite convinced that it was the best treatment for me. He assured me that the side effects would lessen.

As the months passed, so did the need to vomit. Now, I can give myself my shot, hang out with my teenage son (if he'll let me), make a family dinner, and have a good night's sleep—it all seems so normal that once the injection is over, I hardly remember it's shot day.

Tips on Your Injection

○ Pick a comfortable place and a quiet time for your injection. Play music, even listen to the news in the background. Avoid other distractions: tell your family that you'll need to be left alone for a while, don't answer the phone, and so on.

○ Wash your hands with an antibacterial soap and wipe the site of the injection a few times (for comfort) before beginning the process.

○ If you are injecting yourself, you will have been cautioned about air bubbles in the syringe. You may notice some small air bubbles in the pre-filled syringe. To eradicate bubbles, tap gently but firmly on the syringe, using a pen or ruler. Make sure you have a bright enough light to see the bubbles. Tap until the bubbles disappear and you can proceed safely with your injection.

○ Inject more slowly than you were taught to avoid excessive bleeding. Another way to avoid unnecessary bleeding is to withdraw the needle a little more slowly than you might like (this also lessens post-injection pain).

○ If you are on Avonex, your injection is a little tougher, so it's good you need to inject only once a week. An IMD injection uses a 1½-inch needle. You will probably find that your buttocks will be the least painful injection site. Don't worry—you won't have to become a contortionist to inject yourself on the butt. You merely inject higher on the rump, rather than lower. Pulling the skin taut with your free hand will help ease the needle in with the least pain and most efficiency.

○ Over time, learn the injection rhythm that works best for you and your body. You'll be surprised and even impressed by how a few months will bring you to an expert level of knowing how to manage your injection successfully. Believe me, you will feel triumphant.

Of course, if you truly suffer impossible post-injection symptoms, you should talk to your doctor about the pros and cons of changing your medication. But there are ways to alleviate the symptoms, and it may be worth it to you to hang in just a little bit longer.

Coping with side effects successfully

Most doctors, as well as the companies that manufacture the medications, recommend that you eat a meal an hour or so before your shot. Hunger may make you feel weak or fatigued, which won't help you do your best job giving yourself your shot. In addition, having eaten a while—but not immediately—before your injection may help you avoid feelings of nausea afterward.

Another good preventive measure is to take two tablets of an analgesic, ibuprofen, or acetaminophen *fifteen minutes before* the injection and four hours after. This may forestall headache later. (I discovered that taking one Alka-Seltzer tablet before the injection helped lessen both nausea and headache.)

Regardless of which side effects you have, if they persist or seem to worsen, consult your physician.

IN A SENTENCE:

> *Disease-modifying treatments have been proven to help the immune system fight MS and can slow the progress of the disease.*

Think Wellness

IT'S TIME to strike the word "disease" from your vocabulary. Your mission is to be well and stay well while living with MS. So, think wellness. "Wellness" refers to the attitudes, goals, and dedication you bring to your treatment and how you manage your condition on a daily basis. As Dr. Edward A. Taub, author of *The Wellness Rx,* says, "Health is determined primarily by personal responsibility, self-value, and reverence for life."

Wellness is a recognized medical concept that not only acknowledges but insists upon the necessity of full patient participation in the treatment. After generations when patients deferred meekly to doctors, feeling their physicians controlled their fate and deferring to everything their doctors said, this is good news.

Traditionally, Western medicine has had a disease orientation, with the underlying principle that all that is possible is to minimize the physical impact of symptoms and deterioration. On the other hand, a wellness orientation presents the possibility of achieving the benefits of maximum good health—even in the face of a chronic condition. For instance, you practice wellness when you take any of these steps:

○ Modify your diet
○ Increase your level of physical activity
○ Make time in your schedule so that you can rest
○ Eliminate a negative habit, such as smoking, drinking too much coffee or alcohol, or even watching too much television

Since one way of minimizing the return or increase of MS symptoms is to find constructive ways to manage the stresses in your life, it goes without saying that maintaining a wellness attitude will help you in your quest for health in more than one way.

Incorporate wellness into your life

You can integrate the concept of wellness into your life by taking steps such as those listed above to change your physical world, but wellness also has to do with your emotional state. Sometimes the two go hand in hand, as taking up a new activity leads to a greater sense of well-being.

In my own case, acupuncture is one means by which I practice wellness both physically and emotionally. I started seeing a board-certified internist, a man who uses Eastern and Western medical practices, for regular acupuncture treatments.

After noting my inability to relax during the initial sessions, my doctor said, "Your real issue is that you can't stop thinking."

I asked, "How can anyone do that?"

He replied that it took practice, just like learning to play an instrument or learning a new language. My doctor suggested I learn to not-think by listening to calming music on headphones during our sessions. As a matter of fact, he gave me some CDs he had burned himself. I have since discovered that classical music helps clear all those thoughts out of my brain for the half hour in his dimly lit room, and that chants work particularly well.

Now I look forward intensely to my acupuncture appointments. The procedure is an example of wellness in action and the relaxed frame of mind in which I leave the doctor's office illustrates the benefits of wellness thinking.

For a very different route to a similar destination, let's look at what happened to Shalaylah after she was diagnosed with MS. The survivor of an abusive childhood, Shalaylah had always thought that if there was a problem, it was probably her fault. Confronting the news of her MS, she fell into her familiar pattern and thought, "What did I do to make that happen?"

Fortunately, Shalaylah knew she had to keep her mind from running to such bad places. Her solution was to begin taking boxing lessons at her gym. Concentrating on landing a punch or defending against one quieted her mind to a point where she was thinking only of the moment.

As she felt energized physically by her new workouts, Shalaylah also discovered that her tendency to blame herself weakened. Whenever she fell back into thinking she must have done something to cause her MS, she stopped herself and said "You didn't do anything. A situation went wrong. Don't blame yourself. Just fix it."

Boxing helped this woman redirect her thinking and strive toward wellness, just as acupuncture has helped me. Something else could work for you—just keep exploring the options around you. As you do, remember that there will be days when your MS makes you feel lousy, when the positive feelings of wellness seem far away. Rest assured that this happens to us all, but focusing on wellness should always remain a goal. Here is the wellness thinking on that front: Achieve your goal when you can, don't punish yourself when you can't.

Become a peace agent

The late actor Christopher Reeve lived a challenging and ultimately triumphant life, and though he has now passed away, he left a legacy of support for all of those who suffer various infirmities. During his years as a quadriplegic, Reeve continued pushing himself in physical therapy and tried to stay in the best possible condition. About five years after he was paralyzed, he achieved a level of mobility in his pinky—this amazed and gratified his doctors, since such recovery of sensation and motion usually occurs only during the first year of paralysis.

In an interview with Terry Gross of *Fresh Air,* Reeve spoke about the need to avoid emotional paralysis. He also advocated becoming a "peace agent," someone who tries to stay serene and not get riled up by the things life sends our way. These statements are extraordinary examples of emotional wellness, and of wellness thinking, from an extraordinary man who could have quit long before he made them. The title of Reeve's second memoir (the first was *Still Me*) is *Nothing Is Impossible*. Clearly, he lived by these words, and the actor's wellness thinking and doing helped improve the quality of his life and extend his life span. His memoir is a book to take inspiration from, as is our memory of him. His clear message always was do not give up, and he never did, advocating ceaselessly for stem cell research on Capitol Hill, on television and radio, and in many public forums, no matter the personal difficulty of such ventures. Follow his example, fight for yourself and for all of those who cope with MS. A wellness attitude goes beyond simply making the connection between mind and body in treatment to include the emotions and the spirit. It is through considering all four of these components of the self that you can achieve your best health. This is done through productive medical treatment, increasing your energy levels, pursuing a greater level of harmony in your relationships and activities, and establishing an overall sense of well-being in your life.

IN A SENTENCE:

Wellness is another way to expand your lines of defense and expand your view of how to live life completely.

learning

Relapses and Exacerbations

BY NOW, you're aware that MS is a mysterious illness. You've mastered difficult concepts about the immune system, demyelination, and the like as you've learned more about the disease. The vocabulary around the condition is also extremely confusing, which doesn't make it any easier for you, your family, and your support network to understand what you're confronting. Now it's time to get the lowdown on two other terms you need to know: relapse and exacerbation.

A relapse refers to an onset of symptoms to an aggravated degree and for a longer period of time. The symptoms are ones that you have experienced in the past.

When that set of symptoms ceases to be a major part of your life, you have a **remission**. It is important to note that in this case, remission does not mean remission from the disease itself (as the term is used, for example, with cancer), but from the relapse you were having. Just why remission occurs is highly debated and involves many variables, including how well the person cares for himself or herself, how much he or she incorporates rest into managing a relapse, the possibility of

remyelination (regeneration of myelin in certain cells), and the possibility of spontaneous remission.

Two other terms that some doctors and some people use synonymously with relapse are *attack* and *episode*. While different terms may be used partly because the course of MS—and its treatment—vary so much from one person to another, it certainly doesn't make understanding the disease any easier. (In this book, the words "attack" and "episode" are used infrequently, but as a synonym for "relapse" you need to be aware of them in case your MS specialist or any other health-care professional you consult uses them.)

An exacerbation refers to the appearance of a brand-new sign or symptoms.

Exacerbation is also defined as the clinical worsening of signs or symptoms that had been stable for the previous month and that have now reappeared and persisted for a minimum of twenty-four hours. For example, you have weakness in your legs. After you take a warm shower—perhaps too warm—you find that the weakness has increased. If the weakness in the legs lasts for a day, it is an exacerbation, not a relapse (in this particular case, it might be avoided by being very careful of your relationship with heat).

You may be asking yourself, How does this differ from a relapse? As most people use the terms, this second type of exacerbation varies from a relapse in that things get or end up a little worse than they were before.

Signs of an upcoming relapse

Physical therapists who work with MS patients report that there are two major signs that a relapse may be coming on. The first is the feeling of fatigue. The second is a heightened sense of vulnerability, as if the person can tell that something bad is going to happen.

What if you feel vulnerable a lot of the time since you've had your diagnosis? Of course, you don't want to then worry that the feelings themselves will induce a relapse. The main thing to do here is to regulate the stress in your life. Those who keep as much stress as possible out of their lives, and who don't let the remaining stress "get" to them, do better in containing and managing MS.

There has long been speculation that a few medical situations might increase the chance of having a relapse. Immunizations (such as flu shots), surgery, and anesthesia have all been identified as possible culprits.

However, there is no proof that any of these events will induce a relapse. If you find yourself facing such a situation and have concerns, talk them over with your MS specialist or your internist.

Treating relapses

Besides relearning how to best cope with stress, there are other ways to avoid relapses. Stay out of situations that can make MS worse, such as extreme heat. Try your best not to pick up viral infections, and if you do get one, treat it immediately.

Relapses are categorized as *mild, moderate,* and *severe.* If you are having a relatively mild relapse, you may not require any drug treatment. Nevertheless, it is generally not considered a good idea to try to "work through" a relapse. Trying to do this may, in fact, slow the process of recuperation. Many MS patients have found that it's better to rest while they are recovering. It is also wise to avoid engaging in any strenuous activity during your recuperation. In addition, avoid the heat, eat healthily, and stay calm and rest.

Moderate to severe relapses often require steroid therapy. The steroids used to treat MS are cortosteroids and have nothing to do with the steroids athletes use to enhance performance. Cortosteroids are similar to the hormone cortisol, which is produced by the adrenal glands to manage the body's response to stress. This is why cortosteroids work so well in moderating an MS relapse. Steroids help you recover from a relapse more quickly, and they may reduce the chances of further relapses.

Once again, steroid treatment therapies vary widely—from patient to patient, doctor to doctor, and even geographically (some are more popular in one region than another). Cortosteroids can be taken orally (cortisone, prednisone, and decadron) or injected (hydrocortisone and methylprednisolone). ACTH, or adrenocorticotropic hormone, is another drug that is sometimes used to treat relapses; it stimulates the release of cortisol in the body.

Most people tolerate steroids well. Some report feeling better—even euphoric—on them. Most of the immediate side effects of steroids can be dealt with successfully and easily: insomnia is treated with a mild sleeping pill, and an upset stomach or digestive problems can be managed with the aid of an anti-ulcer medication.

However, the problem with steroids is that over the long term more severe side effects appear. Chief among these is permanent bone loss. In addition, with long-term use, steroids may cease to be effective in treating MS. As a result, long-term use of steroids is not recommended.

During your first year of living with MS, if you have a moderate relapse, you may opt to skip steroid treatment. If you are relatively symptom-free, the chances are you will recover from the episode and return to your normal health status. If this does not happen, trust your doctor if he or she thinks treatment with steroids is right for you.

Keep in mind, nevertheless, that as the years roll by, you will be less likely to make a complete recovery on your own from a relapse. Then steroids will become an important treatment option.

IN A SENTENCE:

> *Cope with relapses by knowing what causes them, avoiding situations that may provoke them, and considering treatment with steroids when necessary.*

Making Daily Life
Easier to Manage

AS WITH every aspect of MS, how your condition affects
your day-to-day function will vary according to the severity of
your symptoms. You may have to make only a few adjustments
for ease and comfort in life, or it's possible that you face the
prospect of making major changes in how you make it through
the day. Whatever your situation is, there are plenty of tiny ways
to simplify your daily routine.

Looking good, feeling good

Taking care of yourself helps you to maintain a positive self-
image, and, as you know, positive attitudes are vital in managing the stress that can trigger MS symptoms. You should
continue to take good care of yourself by paying attention to
what you wear, maintaining good hygiene, and sticking to your
grooming rituals.

At the same time, you want to keep things quick, easy, and
simple. One thing that might help right now is to clean out your
clothes closet. Cull out any garments you have not worn for

more than a year (chances are you're not going to wear them again). Get rid of anything you find uncomfortable. Clothing that takes a lot of work to get into and out of—such as items with many buttons and fasteners—are best thrown out as well, unless they're personal favorites.

You can pass these garments along to family or friends, or donate them to charity.

While you're cleaning your closet, check the sock drawer. Get rid of all single socks now. For the future, consider buying the same type and color of sock in bulk to avoid the singles problem.

Don't wear the same thing every day. Vary what you wear to help improve your mood.

If you can avoid ironing, do (don't forget the heat). Perhaps another family member might iron the clothes you need ironed or, if you can afford it, have such garments taken care of by a dry cleaner. Wear cotton as much as possible, and if you do have sensitive skin, definitely avoid heavy wools as well as polyester.

Speaking of dry cleaning, many such establishments in urban or suburban areas will pick up and deliver for little or no charge. Take advantage of such services—cutting down on running such errands as trips to the dry cleaner is a great way to simplify your life.

Get help organizing

There is a wonderful organization called the National Association of Professional Organizers (NAPO). This is the number one group in the country devoted exclusively to getting you organized in whatever areas you feel you need organizing, from your office and your kitchen to your bathroom medicine cabinet, your closets, and your teenager's study areas. When you go to their site online and give them your ZIP Code, they will send you the names of six or more NAPO members in your immediate area.= The members are dedicating to enhancing the lives of their clients to teaching new organizing skills and systems that will streamline the process of staying organizing. Their goal is to help you *take control* of your environment—something I found extremely helpful and that gave me a sense of strength and inspiration when I was stumbling through my first weeks of living with MS.

For example, the woman with whom I worked helped me organize my bills and apply to my insurance company for reimbursement, at a time when all those medical receipts were overwhelming.

You can contact NAPO at www.napo.net/about_napo/ (see Resources, page 247).

Tips on dressing

- ○ If your manual dexterity is impaired, avoid clothing with buttons.
- ○ Want to wear a favorite cardigan or button-down shirt? Simply leave most of the buttons unbuttoned, except for two or three, and treat the shirt or sweater like a pullover.
- ○ If you have some difficulty tying your tie, but can still do it well enough, try loosening the knot without undoing it and pulling the tie over your head. Store the tie that way for next time. Do this on a daily basis and soon you'll have a collection of ready-tied ties for your convenience.
- ○ If tying shoe or sneaker laces is unduly difficult for you, give away the footwear or store favorites for special occasions. Replace shoes with loafers and other slip-ons and look for sneakers that fasten with Velcro.
- ○ When your shoes are wearing down at the heel, have them repaired or buy new ones. Remember that walking correctly is important for your health—you want to preserve your proper gait and not damage your back.

Tips on grooming

- ○ If you have numbness in your hands, buy a spray deodorant and skin cream—they're easier to apply.
- ○ Use massage gloves in the shower or bath to apply soap. You can buy them for about three dollars at most drugstores, and as you wash yourself they will also give you a good circulation massage.
- ○ Get a traction mat for your shower.
- ○ Don't shave in the shower.
- ○ Speaking of shaving: Men, if you have issues of balance or eyesight, use an electric razor to shave; it's safer than a safety razor. Women

should also consider an electric razor for shaving the legs and underarms. If you have your legs waxed, discuss the heat issue with your doctor.

Tips on shopping

○ When you need to, replace vital items in your wardrobe, such as clothes for work, your sweatpants for the gym, your underwear, and even your nightclothes.

○ The Internet is a great, easy place to shop. These days, you can buy almost everything online, from physical aids and clothing to groceries and holiday gifts. (It's also a great way to find support groups for MS and do research on your condition.)

IN A SENTENCE:

> *Do whatever you can so that daily life is simple and doesn't waste your energy.*

Managing
Your Symptoms

AS WITH other aspects of MS, the symptoms you experience will be as individual as you are. If two people were diagnosed at the same time with MS, and with the same type of MS, chances are they would still exhibit widely varying symptoms. So don't waste your time by comparing your symptoms to those of others with MS—that's an exercise in futility, one that might make you worry needlessly and increase your stress levels. Instead, keep your eyes on the horizon and deal with only the things that lie on your own particular pathway to health.

Vertigo and dizziness

Vertigo and dizziness are generally defined as sensations of spinning off balance, whether you are standing up or lying down. Vertigo can cause feelings of nausea and even episodes of vomiting. I get vertigo fairly often. I feel a bit sick, but not really sick—which is a lousy state to be in, especially when you feel like a walking water bed.

While the terms are often used interchangeably, there is a difference: dizziness is less severe, causing feelings of light-headedness without further symptoms.

Unlike most of the symptoms covered in this chapter, which have a concrete, physical basis, vertigo comes with a major emotional component, one of fear and even dread. To lose your balance or to become woozy or sick to your stomach, for no instantly definable reason, is scary and uncomfortable (besides being dangerous, if you suddenly should fall). Don't ever forget your vertigo is real. While there is little that can be done to cure vertigo completely, medication and physical therapy can be of some help in controlling it. In addition, adding simple exercises that promote and improve balance, such as stair stepping (see box), to your daily exercise routine and certain yoga poses, such as The Tree, can help to minimize the effects of vertigo. You can also make sensible adjustments in your daily routine, such as getting plenty of rest (fatigue can worsen vertigo) and holding on to the stair railing while going up or down stairs.

Medicines that help include your basic antihistamines. Your doctor may recommend Benadryl or Dramamine to provide relief if your vertigo or dizziness is mild. For more severe cases, one of the benzodiazepines may be recommended. These include diazepam (Valium), clonazepam (Klonopin), and oxazepam (Serax). These medications are used to treat anxiety and can also work to suppress the parts of the inner ear that may stimulate vertigo. Because benodiazeprines are prescription medications, your doctor who will decide whether such a step is necessary. They are all controlled substances, meaning that can be addictive and should be used with caution.

Physical therapy may help you manage your vertigo through teaching exercises that promote balance. In addition, the therapist will help you determine which positional changes make your symptoms worse and then hold your head in those positions for as long as you can tolerate it. This develops tolerance, which results in your increased comfort. (Physical therapy also helps you manage other symptoms, such as spasticity, stiffness, and issues of gait.)

Balancing Act

I HAVE found that simply stepping up on a stair and stepping back down, then stepping up with the other leg and down again, five or ten minutes a day helps me feel more confident about my balance. Doing this while listening to the news or, better yet, some wonderful music makes this useful exercise fun, too.

Fatigue

Fatigue is one of the most common symptoms of MS, and certainly the one most of those managing MS complain about the most. How we experience fatigue varies. Some people with MS find they are only marginally affected by fatigue—these are often the ones who were in shape and exercised regularly even before their diagnosis. Others complain of simply feeling a loss of energy now and then. A third group complains of persistent and pervasive fatigue. And still others feel tired when they attempt even a limited amount of exercise.

Feelings of fatigue can be placed in two broad categories. There is the simple tiredness referred to earlier. For instance, you might start out on a walk filled with energy, but then you very quickly begin to tire and to feel your legs growing heavy and your steps slower, with a possible dragging of the feet. Once you sit and rest for a brief time, you'll feel yourself ready to go again.

The other type of fatigue manifests itself as an overall feeling of exhaustion. This fatigue lasts longer, is more pervasive, and can limit activity severely from time to time.

Keep in mind as well that, if your diagnosis was accompanied by depression, your depression may contribute to your feelings of fatigue. Depression and feeling tired go hand in hand.

As usual, you are the best judge of how severe your fatigue is and of what helps you cope with it best. A good strategy to avoid fatigue, or to ensure fewer and milder bouts with fatigue, combines exercise and rest. Your fitness regimen should include exercises that work both to promote endurance and to maintain basic mobility. Don't stint on rest or relaxation —these periods do immense work to revitalize you.

Lassitude is a type of fatigue characterized by a feeling of overwhelming drowsiness. Since it is most likely biochemical in nature, medications that alter brain chemistry may be effective treatments. Talk to your doctor, who may prescribe you a drug such as Symmetrel (amantidine), which affects the CNS and is an antiviral medication used to combat fatigue in MS, or antidepressants like Celexa, Prozac, Paxil, and Zoloft, which help combat lassitude and are worth considering for this reason, even if you are not depressed. Stimulant medications, such as Ritalin and Dexedrine, must be used with caution because they are habit forming. Sometimes a well-planned nap and a cup of coffee afterward will do the trick as well as anything.

Here are some tips that may help you keep your energy and any fatigue at bay:

O Do your best to plan ahead. Try to space out strenuous activities and adjust your workday to intersperse strenuous tasks with others that are pleasant and require little expenditure of energy.

O Set your priorities, and make sure you set the right ones for you. This is the time in your life to reconsider old priorities and reevaluate what really matters to you, what you really need, and what you really want. Some of the things we do that we consider priorities in fact may just not matter all that much. Now's the time to shed these false priorities and replace them with real ones (taking care of your own health being foremost among them).

O Make rest part of your daily routine. You'll have to learn to pace yourself. If you've always been a person on the move, train yourself to be more tolerant of inactivity.

When I was first diagnosed, I fought the idea of taking a rest with every fiber of my Type A personality. But as I have continued to talk to others with MS and to adjust to my own situation and my needs, I have found that rest is a great remedy. I no longer see a half hour's rest or snooze as an indulgence but as an excellent therapy aid that increases my energy level and productivity.

Vision changes

Vision changes are one of the most common symptoms for those dealing with MS. Proper vision depends on being able to accurately convey what the eye is seeing to the brain and then relay it to the strong muscles surrounding the eye that are responsible for controlling eye movements. Both of these aspects can be affected by the demyelination that occurs in the CNS when someone has MS.

When the optic nerve is affected by demyelination, optic neuritis can result. This can cause an overall loss of vision, though this loss is usually temporary. If the problem is severe enough, intravenous cortisone is often used to reduce the inflammation. Not all cases of optic neuritis necessitate such extreme treatment, and it is generally advised to take a slow and measured approach to treating this problem. While it can be scary, it usually does resolve itself on its own. When vision improves, it may remain imperfect. The most common problems people notice are the appearance of lighter colors as being washed out and the sensation of having holes in one's vision caused by certain areas of what you are looking at being obscured.

When the muscles of the eye are weakened, the eyes have a harder time working together in a coordinated fashion, and you may experience *double vision (diplopia)*. Extreme cases may be treated with steroids. For moderate cases, you may have to wear a patch over one eye. In less acute cases, the brain tends to learn to compensate on its own. Wearing eyeglasses that have prisms in them may also help the eye bring the images together and resolve your double vision.

If you experience symptoms of vision loss or changes in vision, install night-lights in your home and use them. This will keep you safe and add to a sense of security. In addition, make sure that you have adequate lighting at home and in your workplace. Poor lighting never helped anyone's eyesight.

Spasticity

Spasticity tends to occur in a specific group of muscles, usually the antigravity or postural muscles, responsible for keeping you reasonably upright. These muscles include those in the calves, thighs, buttocks, and groin. Occasionally, muscles in the back may be involved. After spasticity, some stiffness often occurs in the affected area.

The ways of relieving spasticity are similar to those involved most often in successfully relieving related symptoms, such as weakness. They include exercise, especially stretches and other exercises that promote flexibility, and an anti-anxiety medication. It's important to avoid infections, which can aggravate spasticity. In some cases, when spasticity is difficult to manage, mechanical aids such as an ankle-foot orthotic may be necessary.

Weakness

While weakness is a symptom of many other illnesses, if you have MS and are experiencing weakness, it is due to damage incurred to the central nervous system. As a result of your injured CNS, the transmission of electrical impulses to muscles, particularly in the extremities, is inhibited, and that area of the body will feel weaker.

Weakness is inextricably linked with fatigue and spasticity for people with MS. To look at this connection in a positive way, the less stiff (spastic) your muscles are, the less energy you need to expend for any particular movement and the less fatigued you will be—therefore you will experience less weakness.

To combat weakness, you will need to increase your strength and monitor your expenditure of energy. However, exercising to the point of fatigue will not help you. It can be difficult to judge what form of exercise and how much works for you in staying strong. Although there has been some debate over the use of free weights to limit weakness due to MS, experts now agree that thoughtful use of free weights—initially, under the instruction of a trainer—is good for overall strengthening, and this, in turn, helps to minimize weakness. You can work with free weights at home or in the office. After starting with three-pound weights, I've worked my way up to ten pounds; I'm stronger now than when I was diagnosed. There is nothing like increased strength to make you feel more confident.

A reasonable regimen of aerobic exercise, such as working out on your exercise machine of choice, is the best recommendation for management of weakness. In extreme cases, muscles that go unused will atrophy. So, do keep exercising, but be practical about your exercise choices. Keep in mind that by exercising your muscle groups that are still strong, you can support your weaker muscles.

Tremor

There are two types of tremor. The first is wide oscillations, also called gross tremor. The other, which is barely perceptible, is fine tremor. Tremor is most likely to affect the limbs, but it can occur in the head, neck, or trunk, and it can even affect your speech.

Some tremors may occur at rest, but others occur only when you are moving. Most tremors are simply annoying, but some may become disabling. As with many other symptoms of MS, tremor may affect mobility; it can affect balance and coordination as well.

The medication you're taking for other symptoms may also help in controlling your tremor.

Numbness

Numbness is a catchall word that refers to changes in the sensory system that alter sensation. These changes affect the skin most of all, especially on the lower legs, feet, and hands. But it may also be felt as a band encircling the waist or chest area.

Like tremor, numbness is a symptom that tends to be more of a bother than something that will cause you some disability. When it bothers you, therefore, remind yourself frequently that it is annoying rather than disabling.

Keeping fit with exercise is the best medicine for keeping numbness to a minimum. Focus on exercises that help maintain good circulation. A workout on an exercise bike for your legs or on a rowing machine for your upper body will aid in maintaining good circulation. Even a brisk walk will help keep numbness at bay. Here are some other things MS patients suggest doing to help keep numbness under control:

- Flex hands and feet when you begin to feel your extremities getting numb.
- Once you feel the first telltale tingle that will turn to numbness, change position.
- Shake your hands back and forth to improve circulation and eliminate a bout of numbness.
- When sitting for a long period, shake feet and legs periodically.
- Squeeze a tennis ball or one of those small, squishy flex balls you can purchase at almost any drugstore.
- Purchase a Theraband (available at a sporting goods store or online). Learn a few simple stretches you can do with your arms and your

legs. This will increase circulation as well as build strength and maintain flexibility.

○ Don't stay out in the cold too long.

Cold feet

With cold feet, which are related to numbness, once again we have a symptom that is more irritating than injurious to health. The maintenance of skin temperature is an involuntary process controlled by the *autonomic* part of the nervous system, which controls all the bodily functions that happen automatically (heart rate, pupil dilation, perspiration, and the like). Once MS starts tampering with the interconnections of those nerves responsible for the diameter of the blood vessels, the perception of cold feet may result.

You may try rubbing your feet, and that is indeed good for your circulation. Keep in mind, however, that your senses perceive your feet are cold because of nerve damage, not because they actually *are* cold. It will also help to wear warm socks. When you're sitting in a chair reading or watching TV, keep a throw blanket over your feet and legs. The main thing is not to worry. Also, consider this: now, if your boss offers you a promotion, you can say, "I have cold feet, but not about your offer."

Issues of balance and gait

If you suffer severe spasticity or weakness in either leg this will affect your gait and your balance. If these are the symptoms you are most familiar with, you'll want to work on strengthening exercises to strengthen the weakened limb. You might even want to consider an orthotic device for the lower leg to use when the going gets particularly tough. This will help minimize changes in gait; also, because gait affects balance (and vice versa), it will prevent a loss in the ability to balance well.

Quinn was all of twenty-four when she was diagnosed with relapsing-remitting MS. Her symptoms are few, but they tend to involve balance and vertigo issues. "I'm liable to bump into things more than I used to. Sometimes I think people are thinking I'm walking around in a drunken stupor. Then I remind myself that people aren't thinking of me. They're thinking of themselves." When I asked her how she coped, she said she tried all the usual things—exercises, walking more slowly, wearing comfortable walking shoes (her favorite choice was a pair of vintage silver Nikes)—and that her doctor had given her a prescription for clonazepam, which she tried not to take too often. "Mostly," she said, "when I bang an elbow, I just go, 'Oh, it doesn't matter,' and try to forget about it. Sometimes I cry, but I figure that's okay." A little perspective is always good. "A lot of my girlfriends cry much more about this guy or that guy when they've only been dating a few weeks. I'm going to be living with this my whole lifetime."

If you suffer from back pain (whether connected with MS or due to a back injury or any other back condition), you will want to work with your doctor, a physical therapist, or a chiropractor to keep issues of gait from getting worse. This can help to prevent the worsening of your back pain and loss of balance.

When we suffer injury or pain, such as back pain or leg weakness, we tend to compensate for it in how we walk. This only makes matters worse. Take care of any issues regarding how you walk, or gait, due to weakness or pain in any area of the lower body. Don't wait.

A Reflection on "Tingling"

WHEN THE tingling in my calves gets "ugly" and turns to painful prickling, I find the time and a place to lie on the floor and prop my legs up on the wall. Then I close my eyes and practice my own personal brand of meditation: deep diaphragmatic breathing (breath in to the count of five and out to the count of five). I try to empty my mind of all that I can by concentrating on the breathing itself and not the pain. If nothing else, when I get back up after this interlude, I feel calmer, even rested, which at least allows me to cope with the pain better, if it hasn't extinguished it.

While this may not work for you, keep experimenting with pain relief techniques until you find something that does the trick. Remember, your pain is as individual as you are. You are the one who feels it. You are the one who knows it best. And you are the one who will be able to learn and understand what will help most efficiently to relieve it.

Pain

Someone may have already said to you, "At least people with MS don't have to suffer pain." Well, that's one of the biggest myths about our disease. Approximately 50 percent of those who cope with MS experience pain related to the condition at least some of the time. It's thought that most of this pain is caused by short-circuiting in the nerves that carry sensory perception once those nerves have been affected by demyelination in the brain and spinal cord.

The most common type of pain seen in those with MS is often characterized as a toothachey sensation in an arm or leg. I myself describe it as feeling as if you are being punched from the inside out. This kind of pain occasionally occurs in the trunk area. Zostrix, an anti-pain cream, or Neurontin, an antiepileptic medication, may offer relief.

Lhermitte's sign, another form of pain experienced by those with MS, is an unsteady, intermittent electrical sensation that travels down the spine and legs. Often triggered by movements of the neck, it comes on suddenly. Fortunately, after startling you, it passes quickly. While L'hermitte's sign is thought to be a signal of the loss of myelin in the neck or spinal cord region, it is not considered to have anything to do with the course your MS will take.

Trigeminal neuralgia, a severe form of stabbing facial pain, is luckily more rare. This pain is treated with carbamazepine (Tegretol), a medication that "calms" much of the short-circuiting caused by damage to the CNS.

While back pain is often attributed to MS, that may not always be the case. (Just because you have MS doesn't absolve you from the common ailments that afflict everyone.) Therefore, be sure to consult a doctor regarding other health issues that may be affecting your back before attributing back pain to MS.

Simple Ways to Relieve Pain

○ When a little tingle turns to painful prickling, try moving around and gently "shaking out" the limb that's bothering you.

○ If it's primarily your legs that are bothering you, try wearing support stockings.

○ Massage the affected areas with your favorite massage oil. Better yet, try a professional massage. This can help your muscles relax and help you relax, too.

○ Use ice packs on the affected areas.

○ Close your eyes, picture a beautiful view, a person you love, anything positive, and *rest*.

Coping with constipation

Constipation is another thing that people with MS often have a higher susceptibility to. Constipation is defined as the slowing down of bowel motility to the point where it becomes hard to evacuate the stool accumulated in the colon.

The best way to prevent constipation is with diet, which means plenty of fiber in the diet—between 6 and 15 grams a day—and the consumption of lots of water. Foods that are high in fiber include apricots, prunes, peaches, wheat bran, and celery and other vegetables. Vegetables should not be overcooked, since this diminishes their fiber content, which is at its highest when they are raw. The body utilizes fiber best if you drink plenty of water during the day.

It is also important to avoid eating foods that can slow down digestion, such as cheeses, bananas, rice, applesauce, and all fatty foods. Iron supplements may also cause constipation.

If constipation is chronic, bulk-forming laxatives are the next recommended strategy. These include Metamucil and psyllium-seed husks, available under many brand names at your local health-food stores and most drugstores. In severe cases, stimulant laxatives, such as castor oil, may be recommended for short-term use. One cautionary note: stimulant laxatives make constipation worse if taken regularly and can be habit forming. They should remain a last resort and should not be taken without a doctor's recommendation.

Effects on speech

Your speech is controlled by more than one area in the brain. It's easy to deduce then that if you have demyelination in more than one area of the brain, your speech may be affected, if ever so slightly. Demyelination in the *cerebellum,* the area of the brain that controls balance, is the cause of most speech defects. Tremor that affects the lips or tongue may also contribute to speech difficulties.

The most common ways in which your speech might be affected are slurring of words, slowness of speech, and the diminishment of fluency. You may experience one or more of these problems over time. You may also experience something that can best be described as the sense of "tripping" over the tongue.

I try to think I have no speech problems, but sometimes I find one word tumbling in front of another without my wanting it to. Having had some public-speaking experience, I try to rely on my learned skills of elocution: I project my words carefully, pausing for emphasis and the like to get around my galloping words and to slow them down. Nevertheless, I find people don't really notice much. I think it's because very few of us are still capable of speaking the Queen's English in any case.

Anxiety can make any speech problem more apparent. The less seriously you take a slight speech problem, the less anxious you'll be about speaking.

To manage minor problems of speech, pace yourself and pause now and then. Although speech therapy and speech exercises may be recommended and can be helpful, few patients report any long-term improvement.

When the irrational is rational

I have never loved heights, but always attributed this to regular viewings of Alfred Hitchcock's *Vertigo* (I had a crush on Jimmy Stewart). And so, before I was diagnosed, I'd always brush off even the most serious bouts of vertigo—bouts that caused dizziness, nausea, and even loss of balance—to having a thin emotional skin and a big crush long ago. Now I know better: the episodes of vertigo I had were signs of MS.

I've learned a lesson: to trust my symptoms and not to mistrust my reactions to them. Those of us with MS need to take our physical sensations seriously and deal with any symptoms accordingly.

IN A SENTENCE:

> *Knowing more about your symptoms can help prevent them and avoid exacerbations.*

FIRST-MONTH MILESTONE

By the end of your first month, you're beginning to get a handle on managing your MS:

○ YOU HAVE LEARNED ABOUT YOUR MEDICATION OPTIONS AND MADE A CHOICE ABOUT WHAT KIND OF TREATMENT PLAN WORKS BEST FOR YOU.

○ IF YOU HAVE CHOSEN DISEASE-MODIFYING MEDICATION, YOU KNOW HOW TO INJECT YOUR MEDICINE AND HOW TO RECOGNIZE AND DEAL WITH SIDE EFFECTS.

○ YOU KNOW WHAT TO EXPECT IF YOU HAVE A RELAPSE, AND YOU KNOW HOW TO DEAL WITH IT.

○ YOU MAINTAIN A POSITIVE ATTITUDE BY FOCUSING ON STAYING WELL, RATHER THAN BEING SICK.

○ YOU SIMPLIFY YOUR DAILY ROUTINE WHEN POSSIBLE, AND AVOID THE STRESSES THAT CAN AGGRAVATE YOUR CONDITION.

Coping with Stress

NOW THAT you're adjusted (more or less) to your diagnosis and have begun to settle into a daily routine, it's time for a closer look at stress. As I've mentioned earlier, it's important to get a grip on stress, since it can aggravate your symptoms and even trigger relapses or exacerbations.

These days no one can live an entirely stress-free life. Modern life has its built-in stresses, and even a yogi finds it difficult to escape from all of them. Life has its natural crisis points, and then some of us are given a few extraordinary crises to cope with as well—a diagnosis of this unpredictable condition known as MS, to cite the most prominent on your mind right now.

Predictable points of stress

Certain life events and transitions have been shown to cause the greatest stress. They include the death of a child, a spouse, a parent, or another loved one; losing a job, or even changing jobs voluntarily; moving; marriage or divorce; a catastrophic accident or a national tragedy; caring for a seriously ill child or an elderly parent; and of course, coping with a chronic illness, such as MS.

Life is admittedly hard without such events, but sooner or later, one or more of these life crises is inevitable. The best thing to do is to come up with your own system of coping well with stress and pressure. When faced with one of these stressful life changes, try to cut yourself some slack: recognize that you're under stress and don't let the little things affect you—you have enough on your plate already.

If you find yourself having trouble coping with a life-altering event, seek counseling.

Don't panic

The other day, I was watching the news and noticed that my vision seemed blurry. My first thought was that I was having double vision and that the problem was MS related. Then I looked away from the TV to test my eyes elsewhere. The room wasn't spinning. I saw it and its contents clearly, with no blurry vision. No objects that were still seemed to be moving.

The blurriness on the TV screen was just a bad feed, a bad signal. It wasn't me.

Keep in mind that you don't have to accept every thought you have. Take the time to evaluate everything when you're confronted with something stressful. Rushing forward into a panicked state can increase your stress levels unnecessarily. If you slow down and examine the situation, you may often find, as I did with my vision that day, that there is no reason to panic.

There are things you can't control

I live in downtown Manhattan, about a mile from the World Trade Center. On the morning of September 11, 2001, I had accompanied my son to his school (a few blocks farther downtown) and I was walking my dog. Suddenly, this bright and ordinary morning became a day unlike any other in American life.

That Tuesday, and in the days and weeks that followed, people exhibited all kinds of emotional reactions: grief, paralysis, stoicism, depression, etc. Ironically, I stayed on a pretty even keel. Other parents at my son's school and friends around town asked me how I was coping so well. "I've been through a lot," I would answer, without being specific.

I had just lived with the uncertainty of the period of tests and questions prior to my diagnosis with MS; then I had come to terms with and adjusted to my diagnosis. I'm not sure whether these experiences made me stronger, but they certainly made it easier for me to see that there were certain things I could control and others that I couldn't. The terrorism strikes of September 11 were precisely the kind of event over which I had no control. Therefore, I tried not to succumb to unknown fears about whether there would be another attack or whether the ensuing anthrax scares would continue.

I sincerely hope that you are never faced with events such as September 11 as you deal with MS, but the lesson here is clear. It's best to pick up the hand you're dealt and do the best with it that you can. Fearing those elements of life that you can't do anything about will only add to your stress levels. Reminding yourself that fear of the unknown or the uncontrollable can add to stress may help you remain calm during difficult times in your life.

Adapting your attitude

My friend Laura Berman Fortgang works as a life coach. In her book *Living Your Best Life,* Fortgang explains that there are two different ways of looking at the same aspect of your life. "Defining beliefs" can restrict you and box you into preset responses, while "expanding beliefs" can open up new horizons for you. For example, a defining belief would be "I have MS." An expanding belief would be "I am taking care of myself and my new condition. And I am doing a good job."

Looking at these two beliefs side by side, I opted to think of my situation in terms of the latter. Having a positive, expanding attitude will improve your day-to-day life and help to lift the dark clouds from your life. Adapting your attitudes in the direction of expanding beliefs is one way to head off stress before it builds up.

Instead of "I am sick," think, "I am making myself well." And you will do better!

Modifying or lessening stresses

There are obviously going to be times when you can't avoid stress completely. Even though coping with the stress of having MS seems enough to deal with, the stresses of daily life refuse to take a vacation.

First off, remember what is important and don't get worked up or stressed over such things as being late for an appointment or paying your bills, arguing with your children when they start their homework at the last minute, or not being able to find a favorite piece of clothing.

Stress on the job

In 2001, the National Multiple Sclerosis Society presented Gene Fatur with its MS Achiever of the Year Award, recognizing his employer, Turner Construction Company, at the same time. After living for ten years with MS, Gene is still a top-level project manager. He feels that his employer's positive attitude about his ability to work productively has been as vital to his managing MS as the support of his family and the disease-modifying medication he takes. As of this writing, Gene is still on the job. Sometimes he limps a little, but he's also become even savvier about managing his fatigue before it becomes a problem. Given the heightened awareness of employers that "disabled" does not mean nonproductive, Gene's work environment, which he describes as flexible and supportive, is becoming more common in the business world.

Unfortunately, other people with MS don't always have as positive an environment at their job. Take Carla, for instance: an artist, she had been the art director of a food magazine at the time of her diagnosis. Her job was inherently stressful, with many deadlines and long hours; in addition, it involved looking at the results of many photo shoots—not fun, when one of her initial symptoms had been vision impairment. While her vision had improved as she began treatment, Carla did not want to risk any permanent vision loss and decided to leave a stressful work situation. As a freelancer, she has found plenty of work in magazine publishing and more time for her own art, without a lot of the attendant stress from her old job.

If you like your job but just want to reduce the stress levels at work, or if changing jobs isn't an option right now, try to make some accommodations to lower the stress in your workday. Review some of the ideas in Day 6 Living, "Telling Your Employer and Business Colleagues." Here are some more simple tips that have helped others:

○ If you tend to run late, make every effort possible to change your habit. Getting to work on time has as much to do with reducing the anxiety in your life as it has with pleasing your boss.

○ Train yourself not to procrastinate. The anxiety created by leaving work projects until the last minute is one aspect of stress you can at least attempt to control.

○ If you are up to it and don't feel you need a rest, take a walk during your lunch hour. It can help energize you and is certainly good for your overall health.

○ If you get a coffee break (or a cigarette break), use the time instead to go to the bank to avoid the rush at the lunch hour.

○ Don't make plans for Sunday evenings; use this time to rest and prepare for the week.

○ When you are under real pressure to finish an important report or project and just don't have time for much else, lighten up on yourself. The project will get done, and you will get back to your healthy routine.

○ Use business etiquette wisely to lessen the stress of dealing with difficult colleagues or business contacts. Use e-mail whenever possible instead of the phone. If the person starts to press your buttons during a phone call, use reasonable excuses such as "Excuse me, I have to go to a meeting right now," or "Sorry, my eleven o'clock appointment just arrived," to end the conversation quickly.

Stress from running a household

If you've had the primary responsibility for keeping your household tidy and running in shipshape order, it's time to make some changes. Cleaning your house in an all-day session is tiring, and you don't need the stress of worrying what effect that will have on your fatigue level. From now on, try to care for your home in increments, a few tasks or a half hour at a time.

If you have the money, hire a cleaning person to do the heavy work of cleaning, including the kitchen and bathroom. If you need to sacrifice something else in your budget for this, it is probably still worth it.

Also make sure you are getting the help you need from your spouse or partner, and, if they're old enough, your children. Let one of them walk the dog, take out the garbage, or load and unload the dishwasher. As your children mature, assign them more responsible tasks.

Stress in parenting

Every stage of your children's life will come with its own rewards and its own stressful times. They may make you old, but at the same time having kids around will keep you young. While raising children comes hand in hand with its own sorts of stresses—from a child's needy tantrum in public a case of strep throat, from anxiety over whether your child is liked by schoolmates to your dread at his or her being hurt—you can take small, simple steps to manage the stress of parenting.

First, count to ten before you yell. If you don't, a debate with a young, willful, and clever child can often escalate unnecessarily. While we have all heard this advice before, few remember to do it. It's simple, so it's worth a try as a strategy to avoid the old parent-child war.

Don't do it all yourself. If you have the means, hiring a part-time baby-sitter will help you get your rest and keep your temper. Also, if you or your spouse or partner work full-time for a large company, explore the option of taking a family leave.

INFANTS AND TODDLERS

Nap when the baby naps. If you can't nap during the day, trust me, after a year or so of interrupted sleep, this will change. Even a short nap will do wonders to improve your overall attitude and your ability to be patient and enjoy your baby.

Bathe little ones in a baby bath basin in the kitchen sink to avoid kneeling or bending over the tub. If you have to use the tub, put a footstool in the bathroom, so that you can sit while bathing your toddler.

If you are having trouble making sure your baby gets enough breast milk, introduce formula, at least at night. Hungry babies cry.

SCHOOL-AGE CHILDREN

Bathe your child in the evening to avoid adding to the morning rush. If your child wears simple, loose-fitting, non-wrinkling clothing, consider getting him or her dressed after the bath for the next day. It really saves time and fights over clothes in the morning, and nobody knows the difference. And, at least when boys get older, they tend to sleep in their clothes or boxer shorts anyway.

If a child is a heavy sleeper and you walk him or her to a bus stop or to school, get yourself ready before you wake up the child. Your child gets a little more sleep, and you get some time to yourself.

As homework enters the picture, start getting into the habit of having it get finished early in the afternoon or evening. The sooner you start this habit, the easier the future will be. Once weekend homework becomes part of the family picture, begin to encourage your child to get all assignments done by Saturday afternoon at the latest; this saves everyone from the last-minute Sunday blues.

When your junior high school kid wants independence, remind him or her often, but without rancor, that with independence comes responsibility. A cell phone virtually becomes a necessity at this time; help teach your child to report in and to reduce your worries—and therefore your stress.

If your child is applying to a high school or simply going on to an associated public high school, start early. If any additional exams are required, don't hesitate to sign him or her up for a test-coaching course. We all should have had this before we were thrown into the SAT madness. You will be doing your child and yourself a favor. It will lower both of your anxiety levels.

HIGH SCHOOL AND BEYOND

Once children reach adolescence, things get harder and easier at the same time. Here are some tips:

- ○ If you feel that your teenager is having psychological issues regarding puberty, seek help. Many schools have an in-school therapist whom you might consult and who will monitor your child's situation or recommend an outside therapist.
- ○ If things are going relatively smoothly, you may find that your teenager wants to be of help to you and can be a great comfort. Don't lean too hard, but realize you can lean a little. You've been there for him or her, and it's okay for kids to give back.

○ When your teenager learns to drive, make sure a driver's ed class is involved. Don't do it yourself!

○ Start early with college applications. An eager student should be encouraged to start the college essay during the summer prior to senior year.

Stress and dating

There is always stress in the dating process, but it can hurt your health more if you have MS. And a little stress is no reason to drop out of the dating game. Here are a few suggestions regarding dating without too much stress.

When possible, take a rest or nap before an evening out, so that you are on your toes and don't fade too fast.

Don't rush things sexually. If you drink too much on the first date and end up going to bed, you both can be disappointed or embarrassed afterward, and less likely to see each other again.

In general, do not bring up MS on the first date. Consider it a vacation and talk about the rest of your life. The exceptions to this would be if the dating aspect of your relationship had developed after you've known each other and been friends for a while, or if your symptoms are noticeable.

If you realize the relationship is going nowhere, end it gracefully as soon as you can.

When continuing to date one person and becoming comfortable in each other's company, don't wait forever to discuss the future, or ask what his or her intentions are. Better to know sooner, rather than later.

Stressful parents

Most people with MS hope that their parents will be helpful and positive in coping with their diagnosis. But as we've learned, parents can react to the news in a way that's not supportive. If you have parents who can't or won't come through for you, here are some simple tactics to lessen the stress of dealing with your parents:

○ On weekends, screen your calls, and if it's Mom or Dad, pick up only if you want to.

○ If your parents call you late at night, turn off the ringer before you go to bed.

○ If you don't feel able to cope with a family visit at holiday time, make other plans.

○ If you and your family always get together at occasions like your birthday, invite some friends.

○ If things get really rough, ask your specialist if he or she will meet with you and your parents to try to help you straighten things out.

IN A SENTENCE:

> *Whenever possible, avoid the stressful elements of life—but when stress is unavoidable, take steps to reduce its impact on you and your MS.*

learning

Types of MS

AS WITH so much other information concerning this mysterious disease, the experts don't always agree about what the various types of MS are. What follows is as much of a consensus of opinion as could emerge from consulting dozens of texts and websites.

Keep in mind as you discuss your case with your MS specialist and other members of your medical team that classifying the types varies. When you're told you have one kind of MS or another, ask for the criteria. I don't want to confuse you, and the criteria your doctors use in identifying which type of MS you have may not match the standards set down here. In addition, it's important to note that these percentages can vary from study to study. I've tried to use the most universally accepted numbers.

Relapsing-remitting MS

About 42 percent of people with MS have relapsing-remitting MS (RRMS). It is characterized by intermittent relapses when existing symptoms become more severe or by exacerbations featuring new symptoms. In RRMS, full or partial recovery takes place after such incidents. While the symptoms that then occur might be minor and manageable and the disease may seem in remission for months between flare-ups, there often continues to be damage to the axons. Over the course of ten to fifteen years, about 50 percent of those with RRMS develop a more severe version of the disease, **secondary-progressive MS** (see below).

Another form of MS, **benign MS**, is often included statistically and otherwise under the category of relapsing-remitting. People with benign MS may be diagnosed but then, after one or two incidents or exacerbations (usually related to sight or touch), suffer no further effects. If you have been diagnosed with RRMS, there is a complete recovery and no disability. In rare cases, those classified with benign MS may progress to another form of MS, but rarely. Only about 5 percent of RRMS cases are benign MS cases.

Primary-progressive MS

In primary-progressive MS, the disability steadily increases from the moment of diagnosis. People with primary-progressive MS (about 15 percent of cases) often experience difficulty walking or other motor problems at the time of diagnosis. These and other symptoms usually progress slowly and steadily. In the best of cases, they quickly level off, but sometimes the disease will advance.

Primary-progressive MS calls for aggressive treatment.

Secondary-progressive MS

From five to twenty years after a person is diagnosed with RRMS, the disease often progresses to a point where relapses occur more frequently, remission between relapses is never complete, and there is an overall worsening of the person's condition. At this point, the patient can be said to have developed secondary-progressive MS. About 40 percent of MS cases fall into this category.

While it's true that statistics show that most people with relapsing-remitting MS eventually do develop secondary-progressive MS, this finding is drawn from sample populations who did not begin treating MS with newer medication options such as the interferon-based drugs. Most MS specialists feel that within the next decade the picture regarding disability and the inevitability of secondary-progressive MS will be altered radically, as more and more patients thrive with the help of new treatments.

Progressive-relapsing MS

Accounting for 3 percent of cases, **progressive-relapsing MS** is a complex form of the disease. It's very similar to primary-progressive MS, but it includes periods of acute exacerbations that resemble RRMS.

Other terms you might hear about

Chronic progressive MS is a term that you'll find in some MS literature. It refers to the three more serious types of the disease (primary-progressive, secondary-progressive, and progressive-relapsing) collectively, or it can be used as a synonym for any one of them individually.

Relapsing-remitting MS and the chronic progressive forms are together referred to sometimes as **active MS**. This catchall term can include any case of clinically diagnosed MS in which lesions are visible on an MRI and the patient has symptoms and has experienced one or more episodes or relapses.

In the large "Who knows?" department of MS knowledge, **silent MS** ranks right up there. Some people are diagnosed with MS and their MRIs show lesions in the brain, but they otherwise exhibit no symptoms their entire life. These people are said to have silent MS (sometimes called *invisible MS*). Studies have shown that for every four people diagnosed with MS, there is at least one person living with silent MS. With all the advancements in medical testing, it may be possible that some of these cases will be diagnosed in the near future. However, it is to be hoped that they don't end up being treated for something that will never attack them.

The mere existence of silent MS reinforces the fact that so much more research is needed. Why does one person with brain lesions or plaques have symptoms while another with similar lesions has no symptoms for decades and decades? Perhaps lesions in certain areas of the brain and spinal cord affect the larger motor skills and other functions of the body more than lesions in other areas (and people with lesions in those areas develop silent MS).Obviously, if we knew the answer, we'd know more about treating those with the more serious forms of MS.

What MS Is Not

TO SIMPLIFY your conversations with others and to make sure they don't make you more afraid of what you're going through, it is important to realize that MS is easily confused with many other chronic diseases, some of which are far more grave in character.

Here is an example. One day my mother told me about a TV program she'd seen about Stephen Hawking, the great scientist. She was convinced that he had MS. I had to explain patiently that he in fact had Lou Gehrig's disease, or amyotrophic lateral sclerosis. Although sclerosis is in both names, it's an entirely different disease.

MS is not:

○ Amyotrophic lateral sclerosis (ALS).
○ AIDS.
○ Lupus erythematosus, another autoimmune condition, which affects different organs, including the kidneys and the skin.
○ Myasthenia gravis.
○ Sarcoidosis (some symptoms of this disease are similar to those of MS, and the likeness of the word can confuse the uninformed).

Finally, be prepared for one more misapprehension from well-meaning friends and family. People sometimes think that MS is psychologically caused. This is not true. If and when they occur in MS patients, psychological problems are usually the *result* of having to cope with the disease—not a cause of it.

IN A SENTENCE:

> *The sooner you know what type of MS you have, the better decisions you will be able to make about treatment and other changes in your life.*

MONTH**3**

living

Your New Routine

YOUR NEW routine ought to be as similar to your old routine as you want it to be, only better. Choosing which adjustments to make and implementing them may take time. Naturally, your new routine should be individually tailored to your own needs—the changes other MS patients and I have made are merely suggestions. For some who may be able to carry on much as usual, it may be comforting to keep to the same day-to-day routine. Those who are doing just fine may want to adopt a healthier routine to help them in the battle to limit the progress of the disease. Still others who are coping with more than minor symptoms will be compelled to find a routine that helps them cope with and minimize symptoms.

Adaptations can be physical, such as diet and exercise modifications; emotional, such as altering certain relationships; or merely a matter of timing, such as rearranging your schedule to carve out more time to rest.

Adjust your priorities

Introduce any new elements into your daily routine at a pace you're comfortable with. Don't get trapped into thinking that it's some kind of competition and you have to change lots of things overnight.

Here are some adjustments that others have made. My friend Sydney took up yoga and incorporated Chinese herbs into her routine to help her stave off infections and was happy with the results. She also pampers herself as soon as she feels a cold coming on, because she's discovered that it is at these times that she is at high risk of a flare-up.

Mike was diagnosed in his early forties after having serious vision problems, but once he started treatment with one of the disease-modifying medications, his vision returned to normal. Once his health stabilized, he decided to again take up cycling, which he had enjoyed as a younger man. Currently, he's training to ride in a fifty-mile race and is quite happy with his increased strength and endurance.

In my own case, there were some obvious adjustments to make in order to adapt to my new situation. For instance, I had to make room in my life to give myself a shot once a week, allowing adequate time as well to recuperate from any side effects. I also had to have my blood drawn more frequently, to check for any possible effects on my overall health due to the new medication.

With all these extra demands added to my schedule, I saw that the best I could do with the rest of daily life—raising my child, caring for my family, working, and attempting to squeeze in a few visits to the gym each week—was to maintain the status quo. This was not going to be the year in which I would embark on any ambitious new projects. There wasn't much free time to go around, but I did need to rest or nap as well.

Like most people who are recently diagnosed, my hardest emotional adjustment was accepting and dealing with the truth that I had MS. But there were two other feelings that were at the forefront of my emotions: trying to free myself from guilt when I needed to rest or nap, and trying to manage the stresses that continued to upset me.

One final adjustment I made was picking up a new pastime: knitting. Knitting relaxes me and it helps improve my powers of concentration. What began as a distraction soon after my diagnosis has become a true hobby and joy. I've discovered some fabulous new knitting stores and explored knitting with a variety of beautiful and exotic yarns. I've become quite the scarf expert but have maintained my distance from more complicated efforts that involve sleeves, thumbs, or heels. An added benefit has been the beautiful bounty I create each year to give as holiday gifts.

Whatever your interests and talents, from watercoloring to bird-watching or building bird houses, pursue it and you will add a creative and meditative activity to your life that can limit stress and help keep you calm.

Make time for your first checkup with your specialist

If you have a neurologist who specializes in MS, this is about the time you will be scheduled for your follow-up appointment. At this appointment, you will have an examination similar to the one you had when you were diagnosed. Your doctor will evaluate your symptoms and try to evaluate how your treatment program is working. Issues you will want to discuss include:

- How your medication is working for you.
- How you are coping with side effects of the medication.
- How you are adjusting personally to your diagnosis. Do you need some help dealing with your own attitude? Have family issues or relationships been affected? If such problems are bothering you and you don't have a mental-health professional on your medical team, this may be the time to ask your specialist for a referral.

Your job

How well have you been doing your job since your diagnosis? Has work been a place to feel proud that you are still very much a productive member of society, or have you had trouble keeping up with your responsibilities? Do you react to the stresses and pressures of your job differently now than you used to? Of course, if all is going well, there's no need to change a thing about your job.

If you see that there are issues to address at your workplace, talk to your supervisor about making some adjustments. Take your daily trip to and from work, for example. If commuting during rush hours stresses you out more than it used to, investigate other options. Maybe you can come in and leave an hour earlier each day, to avoid the worst of the traffic. Perhaps you can work from home one day a week, hooked up to the office through e-mail.

If either the pressure or pace of your job is too much for you now, it may be a good time to begin to look quietly for another position. Staying in a position where you're unhappy will only increase your stress level.

The other situation where you have to seriously consider a major shift in employment is when you have a very physical job, such as carpentry, tree cutting, or even teaching (especially at the elementary school level). You will want to evaluate how well you can currently do the work and how much you still want to and will be able to do it in the future. Teachers, as well as anyone else whose work involves "care" of the public (this includes even airline pilots and train conductors), should consider how safe those they are in charge of will be.

Your social schedule

If you are like most people, there's always too much to do and not enough time to do it. You do get a sense of accomplishment when you take care of personal responsibilities, but if you're feeling overwhelmed, this is the time to weed out your social schedule.

While I was adjusting to the medication, I cut back on my social life. It wasn't that I was pulling back from life. Let's say, I was filling the well— building my resources in order to be in the best emotional and physical shape I could be. I also decided it was time to reduce the time I spent volunteering at my son's school. I didn't abandon the good cause of participating in his education, but I stopped going to those eight A.M. meetings where parents chat and not a whole lot gets done.

The rule of thumb should be: cut what you can, and keep what you want. If you do trim back on social obligations, don't feel guilty. You have a good reason, and any reasonable friend or acquaintance should understand that you may not be able to do as much as you once did. If anyone does give you a hard time, cross him or her off your list.

Your level of fatigue

The most important symptom to treat is your fatigue, since becoming fatigued can exacerbate any and all other symptoms of MS that you have.

Feeling fatigued can also make you depressed, which will not help you deal actively with managing your MS. This is a time to assess the effect fatigue is having on your daily life. If it is having a negative effect on your life in general, bring it up with your doctor.

Speaking of fatigue, during my first months with MS, I discovered that coffee was beginning to affect my digestion negatively. With considerable regret, I stopped drinking it, substituting green tea. I was concerned that the cutback in caffeine might increase my level of fatigue, but that hasn't happened. The minimal amount of caffeine in my green tea is still enough to have that perk-me-up effect and to help ward off fatigue. So don't be afraid of giving up caffeine as another adjustment to your daily routine.

Coping with the Heat

HEAT WORSENS the symptoms of MS. This happens often enough that it even has a name: *Uhthoff's phenomenon* refers to when MS symptoms get worse because of exposure to heat.

Heat can wear you down and cause fatigue. In my own case, I had always done well in hot weather, but once I had MS, I discovered that heat made me anxious and made me tired. After long exposures to heat, my numbness is aggravated and I experience tingling and greater difficulty with balance. Fortunately, resting in cooler temperatures usually does the trick and brings me back to normal.

When you must go out on a hot day, always wear a hat and light colors to reflect rather than absorb the heat. Walk on the shady side of the street whenever possible. If you're out for a day of shopping or sightseeing, duck into air-conditioned buildings as often as you can. Carry what the health-food stores call a "rehydrating facial mist" (a small spray bottle), since refreshing your face and arms with a cool spray can help you escape fatigue.

The art of humor

Laughter is a natural aid in combating fatigue, keeping relaxed, and maintaining a positive attitude. Humor is an art, one that must be practiced. This does not mean taking all that you might be dealing with lightly, but a sense of humor does help reduce stress and add emotional stamina to your repertoire when you try to see the light side of the small problems and hassles life throws your way. This happened to me, for instance, the day I went for my first MRI as I was being diagnosed. I had gone to the MRI facility by myself and I was becoming tenser as I waited for more than an hour. Around that time, a man who was also sitting in the waiting room got up from his chair and came over to me. He asked, "What are you in for?" I didn't quite like his choice of words, but I replied, "I'm having a brain scan. What are you in for?"

"I have a dislocated shoulder," he said. "May I have your phone number?" Under the circumstances, I found the question astounding. Somehow, I had the wits inside me to make a good comeback: "Don't you want to wait to ask that until you see how the brain scan comes out?"

I laughed out loud. The receptionist and staff who overheard the exchange laughed. Even the guy laughed. I realized that life hasn't changed all that much—men will be men, women will be women, and both sexes will have to deal with that. Somehow the stupid joke helped me wait and to remain patient.

A good sense of humor also comes in handy when someone slights you, says something cruel, or even makes a remark that is not as nice or helpful as it first appears. For instance, Helene, a fifty-five-year-old woman who works in TV, met the thirty-year-old girlfriend of a business associate. No doubt intending to be sympathetic, the younger woman said, "Wow, I'm so sad to hear about your medical problems with MS. I want you to know my grandmother had MS, and she lived to be fifty!"

Helene was hurt at first by this thoughtless remark, but she laughs at it now. She realizes that other things matter more, like getting on with her life.

IN A SENTENCE:

> *Even a few small changes to your daily routine can make for a healthier, happier life.*

learning

Diet and MS

AS YOU take it day by day through the third month since your diagnosis, it's a good time to pay more attention to your diet. Let's follow up on the modifications suggested in Day 5 Learning and learn more about the key elements of nutrition and the importance of a healthy, balanced diet for those with MS.

The great nutritional debate

The first challenge we face is sorting our way through the confusing morass of details in the popular and scientific media about what Americans should and should not be eating. Does a particular food ward off cancer or promote heart disease? What is the right amount of protein to eat to ensure healthy bones? Is the best diet low in calories? fat? protein? carbohydrate? There's so much conflicting information out there that you can easily get overwhelmed. The experts themselves don't seem to be able to figure it out either.

There's an added wrinkle that comes with age. Most of us diagnosed with MS over the age of thirty (and plenty of those diagnosed at a younger age) have other health issues that we cope with as well. If we're at risk of heart disease, we already try to incorporate low-fat habits in our daily caloric intake.

Those with high blood pressure limit salt intake. Some of us also manage type 2 diabetes by eliminating sugars and most other simple carbohydrates from the diet. If you are already practicing such dietary modifications, it's realistic to wonder how much more diet modification you can take.

Improving your daily diet, unless it's currently terrible, will have only a limited amount of influence on the course your MS takes. Nevertheless, there are at least two very valid reasons to try to eat the foods that are best for you. First, eating well can not only make you feel better physically but also give you a sense of control over your life. This reinforces the positive attitude that is key to managing stress. Second, if you improve your health through a wise diet, you improve your chances of fighting the disease.

Protein and MS

Protein is essential for good health and is one of the body's cornerstones for good health maintenance. Tissue growth and repair would be unsuccessful without it, and in fact next to water, this nutrient is the major substance in the body, accounting for about half of our dry weight.

Unfortunately, in the past decades protein has gotten a bad name from many health and diet gurus. They have told us that Americans eat too much protein. This well-meaning but wrongheaded advice stems from the fact that we have tended to get protein from animal products, such as meat and eggs, and much animal protein comes with fat.

There are several ways to get the protein you need without eating too much fat. Replace red meat with chicken, turkey, or fish. When you do eat red meat, use leaner cuts of beef. Avoid most cheeses and high-fat dairy products, buying lower-fat or nonfat versions.

Furthermore, not all proteins come from animal products. Tofu is a valuable source of this key nutrient. You can also find it in such vegetable products as beans, whole grains, nuts and seeds, and grits and oatmeal.

When you eat fish, choose among the kinds that are rich in the omega fatty acids (particularly omega-3, -6, and -9). It's important to reiterate that while we seem to be getting the message regarding omega-6s, most Americans still fall well short of the recommended amounts of omega-3s in their diets. Remember to include flaxseed oil and ocean fish in your diet. Your best bets are all types of salmon, albacore tuna, trout, herring, and anchovies. Eating your protein with the omega acids built in is a great idea if you want to follow a heart-healthy diet.

Fat

Fat comes in three varieties, and as you learned in Day 5, it's not all bad. The right kind of fat is necessary in a healthy diet (even if you are managing MS) and it is no longer a dirty word.

Fat is made up of *glycerol* and *fatty acids,* both essential elements in healthy bodily function. The cells of the body use fat to produce many of the hormones vital to the regulation of bodily functions. Fat is necessary for the absorption of the fat-soluble vitamins (A, D, E, and K). It also helps keep the skin and the hair healthy. In addition, the so-called essential fatty acids cannot be manufactured by the body, leaving us dependent on the "good" fats as a source for them.

The three kinds of fat are saturated fat, polyunsaturated fat, and monounsaturated fat. Saturated fats are the "bad" fats, while polyunsaturated and monounsaturated fats are the "good" ones, which perform the vital functions needed to keep the body working. If you're concerned about heart disease, keep in mind that polyunsaturated fats actually raise the levels of good cholesterol in your blood. So concentrate on the good fats and eliminate saturated fats wherever possible. Cut out such high-fat foods as ice cream, most cheeses, junk food, and fast food.

It's important to note that further studies have shown that people with MS benefit from a diet low in saturated fats, particularly animal fat. And, as mentioned earlier, research has also shown that a diet rich in polyunsaturated fats can be helpful to those managing MS.

If you read nutritional labels, you'll see that oils are used in most processed foods. While all oils are a mixture of saturated, monounsaturated, and polyunsaturated fats, some are better for you than others. Safflower, canola, and sunflower oils are the best; try to avoid foods made with coconut or palm oil, or cocoa butter. When cooking, put aside the lard or butter and use one of the three oils mentioned above or olive oil. If you count your calories, keep in mind that fats make up 20 to 35 percent of your daily food intake, and experts recommend that the majority of these be monounsaturated or polyunsaturated.

Another excellent source of good fat is flaxseed oil. You can use it in cooking or in salad dressings. It's also available as a supplement in health-food stores, in capsule form.

There is a theory that those with MS are less able to process fats efficiently, and that this is due to our having a lecithin deficiency. Lecithin (also known as phosphatidylcholine) is a phospholipid, an important component of the cell membrane. Since studies have shown that some people with MS exhibit a marked decrease in the lecithin within the myelin sheath, you may want to consider taking a lecithin supplement.

Carbohydrate

Carbohydrates are a major—sometimes, the major—source of energy for the body. Here again, one type of carbohydrate is not as good as another. Complex carbohydrates—fruits, vegetables, and foods made with whole grains—are essential to include in your diet, in moderate amounts. Simple carbohydrates, such as refined sugar and white flour, should be avoided; these calories have little nutritional value.

The latest guidelines from the Institute of Medicine of the National Academies, issued in September 2002, recommend that carbohydrates make up 45 to 65 percent of your daily calories.

Complex carbohydrates, such as whole grains and the foods made from them, are the best source for fiber. Although it is not a nutrient itself, fiber facilitates the efficient digestion and absorption of the essential nutrients.

Fiber is found in the cell walls of plants: fruits, vegetables, legumes, and nuts. You can kill two birds with one stone by snacking on high-fiber, low-fat crackers, replacing refined carbohydrates and bad fats with fiber and complex carbohydrates; look for brands such as Bran Crispbread, Bran-Crisp, Ryvita, and Wasa.

In general, Americans do not eat enough fiber-rich foods. The American Cancer Society recommends that Americans consume between 20 and 35 grams of fiber a day, but it is estimated that most of us consume only 10 grams daily.

New Tips and Tricks
from the Low-Carb Revolution

I'M NOT a big fan of low-carbohydrate diets, but over the last decade we have learned that carbohydrates are indeed what makes us far. So, if you have a weight problem and want to control it, following a low-carb diet might be the way to go. Check with your doctor first, of course.

Because of the recent low-carb-diet crazes, you have many new low-carb products to choose from while following such a diet, including:

- ○ Men's Bread and Woman's Bread, from French Meadow bakery: these are low in carbs and high in flaxseed content.
- ○ JJFlats Breadflats: total carbohydrate per serving, 10 grams (3 percent of suggested daily intake).
- ○ Tumaro's Gourmet Tortillas: total carbohydrate per serving, 13 grams (4 percent of suggested daily intake).
- ○ LifeStream (from Nature's Path Foods): The LifeStream brand offers a wide range of whole grain pasta products that are made with flax meal, a source of both omega-3 and -6, and are low in carbohydrates.
- ○ LifeStream rotini: total carbohydrate per serving, 36 grams (12 percent of suggested daily intake).
- ○ BioNature organic pasta: BioNature offers 100 percent stone-ground whole durum wheat pasta products; for instance, its elbow pasta has 42 grams of carbohydrate in an average-size portion (14 percent of suggested daily intake).

Having lived with MS for some years now and lived with all the research and information we all get from the Web, our books, our doctors, and our friends, my own personal take is that the best diet is simply this: low-fat, no saturated fat (except for the occasional treat), and low-carb (meaning avoid white flour and sugar); on top of this base, eat plenty of good vegetables (steamed, not boiled) and seasonal fresh fruits. If you are concerned about dairy fat, either cut dairy out or use low- or nonfat products. You may look as far as you want for a diet formula that cures, but this short paragraph may also free you to think you're doing okay and give you time to turn your focus to exercise, so necessary to all of us.

Alcohol

One glass of wine a day may be recommended for heart health and may be consumed by a person with MS without fear of exacerbating symptoms. More than one drink daily may aggravate tremor or vertigo, and too much alcohol will begin to affect your balance and may even lead to falls. Over time, too much alcohol will also negatively affect memory and your brain cells.

If you like wine and had a glass or two more than usual during the time you were going through being diagnosed with MS, this is normal. But once you have accepted your diagnosis, it is extremely important to keep alcohol consumption to a minimum, both for the reasons stated and since alcoholic beverages are generally empty calories. If you feel you are having trouble maintaining moderation, seek help.

Good News About Sugar Substitutes

Not all sugar substitutes are created equal. Certainly, you want to avoid saccharin and aspartame-based substitutes, which are bad for your overall health.

Splenda is one of the new kids on the sugar substitute block. It is a calorie-free sweetener made from dextrose and sucralose (which are considered sugars), without additives.

Stevia Extract is the real new star. It is an herbal extract, made from Stevia Rebaudiana leaves, and is calorie free. This is my personal favorite for both flavor and health.

The importance of variety

Eating should not be boring. Nor should eating well be boring. There are plenty of great food choices out there, so don't think that adapting a healthier diet—and sticking to it—means you're going to have to eat the same bland foods, fixed the same way, day after day. Read up on nutrition, peruse health-oriented cookbooks, watch the cooking shows on TV, and vary the foods you eat. You will discover that you have an array of healthy food options and you can experiment to please your palate and keep meals interesting.

Make your diet choices wisely and make the right ones for you. If you fall off your diet one day, you will not lose all the benefits healthy eating can provide. (And, of course, having a yummy, high-fat, high-calorie snack now and then also makes you feel better—just don't overdo the treats you reward yourself with!) It's what you do over the course of a year, not what you do on one particular day, that counts.

Food Shopping Online and Other Options

THESE DAYS there is a bevy of "Web supermarkets" that offer an almost overwhelming array of low-carbohydrate and low-fat products. Some of these include:

Viva LowCarb Superstore: www.vivalowcarb.com.

Low-carb.com is a site where it's easy to can shop by category. For instance, the bakery section offers many delicious breads, muffins, bagels, waffles, and dessert choices. www.low-carb.com.

Dreamfields Healthy Carb Living: Dreamfields specializes in low-carb pastas that are 65 percent lower on the glycemic index than regular pastas. These pastas also contain no cholesterol or saturated fat.

Your local health-food store can be a great source for healthy low-fat and low-carb foods. Along with other specialty food stores, many health-food stores deliver. If you don't have a good health-food store nearby, my local one, Health & Harmony, has a wide range of choices and delivers nationwide. Its phone number is 212–691–3036.

Diet plans recommended for MS

Given the mysterious nature of MS, it is important to acknowledge that while diet may be helpful in maintaining good health, it cannot in any way be considered a cure for the disease. Nevertheless, there seems to be a consensus that adhering to a healthy diet may improve your attitude toward your condition and, therefore, help minimize symptom flare-ups.

Over the years, several diets have been touted as particularly suited for people with MS. They include the Swank Diet, with an emphasis on low-fat protein; the all-natural Evers diet, which includes wheat germ and many raw foods; the low-fat, gluten-free MacDougall diet; and an allergen-free diet. If you're interested, do the research on them, but by all means talk to your medical team before embarking on one of these, or any other diet.

IN A SENTENCE:

> *Making improvements in your daily diet will help enhance your overall health.*

living

Sex
and MS

JUST WHEN you thought you had all the paradoxes you could carry in your basket of life, here's another. If you are symptomatic for MS, the exertion of sexual activity can cause you pain and stress; sex can briefly exacerbate relapsing-remitting MS. On the other hand, the pleasure of a loving sexual experience can indeed reduce stress. So, what to do? Well, try it—if you don't like it, try it another time; if you do like it, make a point of trying again.

Glib as such words are, the truth is that you're not going to know how to incorporate sex successfully into your post-diagnosis life until you try it a few times. As you experiment here, it helps to have a willing, understanding partner, and to communicate freely and openly about what works and what doesn't.

Over time, you will probably have some problems. The fact is that more than 90 percent of men with MS report problems in their sex lives; for women the figure is 70 percent. Be patient, talk about the problems that arise with your partner, and if you have had a satisfying sex life, you probably will once more. If your sex life has been problematic, you may want to examine why before the hurdles that you're now facing make it

unalterably worse. Keep the lines of communication open with your partner. Consider seeing a therapist or, if your partner is willing, a couple's therapist. If you're comfortable enough to talk about the problems with your
MS specialist, internist, or gynecologist, by all means do so.

Incontinence

Surprisingly, the most common problem in the sexual arena isn't strictly
speaking a sexual one at all. Both sexes report that they often have difficulties with bladder control. The people I interviewed were often embarrassed to mention this, regardless of their age or health status. Both women
and men said they were afraid of losing bladder or bowel control just when
things are getting hot.

Polly's story is typical. She and Ken had been married about six years
when she was diagnosed with MS. Many things were getting in the way of
their sex life: her exhaustion, the rigors of raising two young children, work,
and Polly's need to take care of her own health. Added to those was her fear
that she would "wet the bed," as she put it.

Polly said, "The funny part is, Ken's seen me giving birth twice. I've got
nothing to be embarrassed about, but I'm still . . . well, embarrassed." Polly
knew her embarrassment was illogical, but that was the way she felt.

The good news is Polly and Ken have adjusted to their new situation and
once again have a decent sex life. Polly goes to the bathroom before any
foreplay or just when foreplay starts. Ken knows that during sex Polly may
urgently need to pee again. In most cases, the brief interruption does not
spoil the mood; if anything it enhances it, Polly says, because she feels free
to express herself sexually. Polly advises, "It's good for everyone to keep in
practice. With practice, you may not become perfect, but you do get better."

To cope with incontinence, you and your partner should follow Polly and
Ken's lead, communicating openly and keeping in touch with each other
physically. On a practical level, make sure to use the bathroom before any
foreplay begins.

Problems of sexuality

Technically speaking, sexual response is dependent on reflexes triggered by neural transmissions, which may be stimulated by many different

sensations. Nerves near the base of the spinal cord carry electrical signals from the brain to the genitals. Needless to say, these nerve pathways are highly complex and any problems with the condition of these nerves may short-circuit the transmission of impulses and cause some degree of sexual difficulty or dysfunction.

The level of dysfunction varies depending on the type of MS; for example, relapsing-remitting MS would interfere with your sex life less noticeably or severely than one of the progressive types of MS. Dysfunction also depends on how long you have lived with MS. In the first year, many of those diagnosed with MS report no change in their level of sexual desire or ability to experience sexual pleasure.

As would be expected, sexual problems can vary for women and men with MS.

Problems for women

There are several different kinds of sexual problems that arise for women. Vaginal lubrication may diminish and a weakening of vaginal muscles may occur. Some women report an uncontrollable or reflexive pulling together of the legs during intercourse (the technical term for this, in case you discuss it with a doctor, is *abductor spasms*).

However, the most frequent complaint for women is a decrease in genital sensation. Women also complain of loss of interest and diminished orgasmic responses. Common sense indicates that these two complaints can reinforce each other, making the problems worse. With the expectation of very little joy at the end of the rainbow, who wouldn't lose interest? And with a loss of interest, you are less likely to feel stimulated enough to "go for it."

While some women have this problem with numbness, others experience a heightened sensitivity. They may have uncomfortable tingling and itching in the vaginal area, which makes arousal almost unbearable to even contemplate.

And there are women who are subject to *both* numbness and hypersensitivity. Such was the case with Nancy, who was in her thirties when she was diagnosed. Nancy is in a long-term relationship with a woman named Gemma. During her first year with MS, what had worked for the couple sexually before didn't work for Nancy anymore as she grappled with alternating periods of numbness and extreme sensitivity. Nancy just "walked away" from sex altogether, which naturally caused problems in her relationship. The tension between them grew, until Nancy finally confronted the issue, spoke up, and told Gemma about her physical discomfort.

Nancy had worried that Gemma would think she was making up her symptoms and that her aversion was purely psychological. Instead, Gemma was glad to hear what was wrong, and they were both relieved.

Since Nancy began communicating more about her needs, the two women have managed to reestablish a satisfying sex life. "I let her know beforehand that we have to be prepared to stop at any time if I start feeling that uncomfortable tingling," Nancy says. "I have to warn her. I don't want to disappoint my lover, but I do speak up when the tingling starts, because it goes from uncomfortable to unbearable in no time." As Nancy sees it, they are getting to know each other sexually in a different way, and while foreplay takes longer, there is nothing wrong with that.

Problems for men

The most frequent problem men with MS report is erectile difficulty. This can be caused by anxiety, perhaps even by self-induced pressures you feel during your first year with MS. If the problem persists, talk to your doctor.

Jimmy is a gay man who has been in a long-term relationship for about seven years. He had begun having bouts of impotence even before his diagnosis. Once he was diagnosed, he noticed that these incidents coincided with his flare-ups. Fortunately, Jimmy and his partner have been together long enough that they were not going to let a diminished sex life, in his words, "ruin everything else." Jimmy finally mentioned the problem to his doctor and was given a prescription for Viagra. He now takes a pill a few hours before sex. This means he and his partner have to plan ahead, but as he told me, "After a few years together, doesn't everyone?" What Jimmy is most grateful for is having a committed partner.

On the other hand, my friend Bill still enjoys his sex life with his wife without the aid of Viagra. His disease-modifying drug helps with his energy level and stamina. As he puts it, when it comes to sex, there has been "a slight diminishment, but not a collapse. Let's put it this way. My wife knows how to help and how to be patient, and certainly I can please her in other ways."

Dealing with dysfunction

Any couple who wants the relationship to work should ideally discuss all issues that arise around sex and sexual dysfunction. While it can be embarrassing to talk about things like bladder or bowel control, open communication is a key tool if you are going to continue to have a pleasurable, fulfilling sex life.

No one has a perfect sex life, so forget blaming all of it on MS. You'll only put more pressure on you and your partner. The first thing to deal with is your anxiety about the situation. The best way to lessen that anxiety is to have a positive attitude.

The better you feel, the more likely you are to have a positive sexual experience. And a fulfilling romantic session will make you feel better in turn. So, get comfortable, make sure you are not fatigued, and if it doesn't feel good, or worse, if it hurts, stop and try something different.

Birth control

In most cases, birth control pills are safe for women with MS. You should discuss whether the pill is safe for you with your MS specialist as well as your gynecologist.

More and more experts recommend against the IUD for women with MS, because that device prevents pregnancy by causing a low-grade inflammation of the lining of the uterus.

The condom is always a popular recommendation. Women who go off the IUD or are uncomfortable with taking birth control pills, especially now that there's so much other medication to take, may want to revisit this option with their partner. Another alternative is a diaphragm accompanied by a spermicide—these have not been found to be harmful to women with MS.

If you have had all the children you want to have, or if you have decided not to have children, this is a good time to examine a sterilization procedure: tubal ligation for women, vasectomy for men.

Give yourself time to decide on your choice of birth control, however, since this is your first year, with a whole new picture of health and well-being in front of you. Stick with condoms and diaphragms until you make a long-range decision regarding what you want from your own and your partner's reproductive life.

MS *and menstruation*

Some women who are dealing with MS find coping with their monthly periods to be the same old thing after they've been diagnosed. Others find menstruation worsens their MS symptoms. In addition, those who already suffered from PMS often find that their PMS symptoms become worse.

While everyone's experience is different, most of the women I've talked to in their twenties and thirties found their periods to be pretty much the same with MS as their cycle was before (the exceptions were those who already suffered from fairly serious PMS). A woman who was diagnosed at thirty-two reported that she had normal periods until she was forty-seven and entered menopause.

Fluctuations in hormone levels in the body, particularly levels of estrogen, are thought to be responsible for the direct connections between increased frequency and severity of exacerbations with prolonged bouts of PMS. If your menstrual periods are worse since you've been diagnosed, do not give up hope—your specialist and your gynecologist can help you.

Many women find that going on oral contraceptives offers relief from the symptoms of both MS and PMS. If you're older and this doesn't work, early intervention of hormone replacement therapy (HRT) can help.

If neither birth control pills nor HRT does the trick, a mild dosage of an antidepressant or an anti-anxiety drug can help you through your period.

Finally, some women worry that their vaginal muscles may go so bad that a tampon will fall out after it's inserted. More than one top-notch gynecologist told me this just doesn't happen.

IN A SENTENCE:

> *Communication and trust will help you overcome any obstacles MS puts into your sex life.*

learning

Making Exercise Your Ally

YOU LEARNED a little bit about the benefits of exercise in Day 5 Learning. Now that you've had more time to adjust to your new life, let's focus some more on the relationship between levels of physical activity and your MS.

Being physically active doesn't mean you have to exercise as much as a star athlete or supermodel. The truth is, any physical exercise (as long as it's not injurious) is better than no activity at all.

My mother often speaks of another virtue of exercise. "Stay active," she says. "Depression doesn't hit a moving target." She's right—exercise truly does help your mood. If you can get yourself out for a walk, a workout at the gym, or a swim at the local pool, there are emotional benefits as well as physical ones. Exercise is a quick pick-me-up, no matter what level of motion you are capable of.

If you were already active before your diagnosis, keep at it and you can keep the treasure of a healthy body relatively intact. On the other hand, if you have been inactive, exercise doesn't have to be an exhausting workout or a chore. In fact, you can begin easing into a more active life by striking the phrase "working out" from your vocabulary. Instead, think of exercise as walking for health, stretching for health, and breathing more deeply for health. In short, you do not need to be an exercise junkie to get yourself in better shape. And the better the shape you are in, the more manageable you will find the symptoms of multiple sclerosis. Some of your best allies in living the good life with MS are strength, endurance, flexibility, and balance, all of which are improved with exercise.

Choosing the right sport or activity

The kind of exercise that is safe and enjoyable for you will depend on your symptoms, how frequent your relapses are, and your level of disability. During the first year, many of us experience limited or no disability. However, don't assume that this means that you can continue to pursue your favorite sports with a fervor equal to that of your pre-MS days. Especially if you were involved in a contact sport or other rigorous activity, it is wise to reexamine your exercise plan. The reason is simple: any injury, including a sports injury, can trigger a relapse in people with MS. In that respect, sports where you can fall or collide with another participant—such as biking, in-line skating, figure skating, and skiing—are very risky. In the end, the choice you make will depend on the ratio of your love of a particular sport to your risk of injury, but this may be the time to give up your touch-football league for another sort of activity.

Here are a few safe exercise choices:

Walking. For a number of reasons, walking is the most popular choice of exercise in the United States these days. You don't have to join a health club, and it doesn't require any monetary investment beyond a pair of good walking shoes or sneakers. You can do it with a friend, so you can visit and walk at the same time, and have someone to count on, should you need help. Third, your risk of injury during a brisk two- or three-mile walk is minor. Especially if you've not exercised in the past, all of this adds up to a perfect plan for improving your health and stamina after having been diagnosed with MS.

Swimming. Swimming is an especially good exercise because it involves all the major muscle groups and it is low impact. However, unless you're lucky enough to have your own backyard pool, it can be difficult to find a place to swim, especially in the winter months. Many health clubs and gyms have indoor pools, but if you can't afford a membership, there are lower-priced alternatives. Check the local Y, or ask around since some towns and cities have municipal indoor pools with low fees (sometimes open to nonresidents).

Don't give up. Being in the water is good for you. If you're not a good swimmer, see if your local Y has beginners' classes or water-exercise classes designed for nonswimmers. Even simply treading water in a pool is good for you, far better than sitting around wondering what to do for exercise.

Fitness machines. Home-exercise machines are very convenient and generally a safe way to increase or maintain fitness. A stationary bicycle or a rowing machine, for instance, will exercise your entire body while eliminating the risk of falling.

If you have the space, you may want to purchase a stationary bike or other exercise machine for your home. You save the cost of joining a health club and it's far easier to fit exercise into your schedule. The downside of having a home-fitness machine is that you have to be self-disciplined enough to use it—there's no one but you to see that you use it regularly. Some people report that drawing up an exercise schedule keeps them motivated.

The price of these machines has dropped considerably, and they can be purchased at sporting goods stores, from catalogs, or online.

Aerobics. Aerobic exercise of any kind builds stamina and endurance. If your doctor approves, sign up for a series of classes in aerobic exercise or aerobic dance at your gym, Y, or community center. Make sure you mention your health status as you register and at the first class. No one will turn you down, but your teachers and trainers will want to know, in order to help make you well and not hurt you.

Yoga. The benefits of yoga are manifold, especially for those with MS. Practicing a few yoga poses regularly will help improve your balance and increase your flexibility, thus limiting stiffness and spasticity. Yoga can also improve your breathing and your overall sense of well-being. It can maximize your level of tranquillity while minimizing tension. Sounds almost too good to be true, but it's not!

Many gyms offer classes in yoga, but if you don't already belong to a gym, look around first for a yoga center. Increasingly common in

American cities and towns, they focus more on the central aspect of yoga as taught by the yogis. Classes at such centers or institutes tend to incorporate more breathing exercises, which will help you manage stress, into the physical exercise common in yoga classes everywhere. By contrast, classes at a gym can get caught up in Western notions of competition among students and the quest for excellence.

In any case, another advantage of yoga is that no special equipment is needed and that you can do it at home, at your own pace and on your own schedule. When you start out, a class or two is very helpful to learn the poses the right way.

Weight training. You get a big boost to your strength and your endurance from a regimen of training with free weights. They don't have to be heavy, and you don't have to be a bodybuilder.

If you have problems with balance, an advantage to weight training is that you can simply stand still and lift weights. Lifting weights will not only make you stronger, it will help build confidence, too.

T'ai chi. Although in China t'ai chi is traditionally considered a medicine, in North America it's now widely practiced as a form of exercise and as a relaxation technique. In general, the arms trace circles in the air, slowly and smoothly, while the weight is shifted from leg to leg. As you practice these movements, you also practice breathing techniques. A specific series of movements is referred to as a form. The theory is that t'ai chi balances the opposite forces of yin and yang. For our purposes, it is good enough that t'ai chi is definitely beneficial to your coordination, sense of balance, and level of relaxation.

You can find a t'ai chi class at your health club or your local community center.

Getting started

Once you've picked your sport or activity, the next step in setting up an exercise plan is to consult your doctor. If you're already physically active and want to notch up your regimen, inform your MS specialist what you do, how often, and for how long. If you're just starting out, tell him or her what form of exercise you're interested in. In either case, your doctor can advise you whether your plan seems reasonable. (For example, a plan that involves swimming thirty minutes three times a week would seem reasonable to most doctors, as long as the pool is not overheated, but planning to swim every day for an hour or more would place excessive demands on your body, and increase the chance of injury.)

When it comes time for your workout, always warm up before you exercise and cool down afterward: stretches and other light exercise before and after your workout go a long way toward preventing injury, especially cramps, strains, and muscle pulls.

Pick a reasonable exercise goal. The idea here is to settle on a program for yourself that you feel you may be able to accomplish, whatever that might be. Some people say to themselves, I'm going to change my life; I'm going to exercise every day, and I'm going to wind up with a body like this athlete or that performer. In most cases, these are the people who fail at meeting any goal at all. The point of a goal is to set one for yourself that will challenge you but that is still within reach. For instance, if you have not been exercising, decide to walk half an hour three days a week. If you have been using an exercise bicycle two to three times weekly, increase it to three to four times. These are goals that will help you exercise more; they're not so unrealistic that you will soon give up.

Increase the duration and the difficulty of your workout gradually, in small increments. For example, if you've just taken up jogging and chosen a goal of running three miles four times a week, don't plan on doing this in one or two weeks. You'll need to start out slow, running for a while at a slow pace, then walking to catch your breath, and running again. You may do only one mile the first few times, and you may not be up to running four days a week. Your goal is something to build up to, not something you've already achieved. Be patient with yourself. It's not a competition, and the only race you want to win is the one of good health.

Finally, if you are injured, don't neglect it. Even something that seems like nothing, such as a muscle strain, can aggravate your MS. Consult your doctor as soon as you feel pain, minor or major. Stop exercising until he or she gives the go-ahead. Don't take any injury lightly—take care of it before it gets worse.

Staying motivated

In all aspects of life, motivation is the key that unlocks the door to success. This certainly holds true for beginning an exercise program and then sticking with it. While you may start strong, filled with conviction and ready to charge full speed ahead, motivation is a tricky thing to hold on to. It eludes all of us at times, and you have to find it again and grab hold of it. Here are a few helpful hints to get you motivated and keep you motivated.

○ Set goals you can achieve. If your aims are unreasonably high, you may be more tempted to give up.
○ Unless you are sick or injured, work out regularly.
○ If injury, fatigue, or relapse causes you to not exercise, try not to lose all the benefit you've gained so far. You will probably still be able to perform a series of simple stretches: flex your hands and feet, lift your arms up, and lift your legs up. Do what you can to stay in the exercise game.
○ Be creative in working your way around obstacles to exercise. If you think you don't have time, make time. If you think you don't have a safe place to exercise, join a gym. If you don't have the money to join a gym, ask for a gift membership for your birthday.
○ Make stairs your ally. If you have a two-story house or apartment, don't save time by minimizing the times you have to go up and down stairs. Take extra trips. It's exercise. At work, don't take the elevator. Take the stairs. In this case, more is healthier—but make sure you hold on to the banister for support!
○ Look at the big picture. If you're not ecstatic about the progress you've made in a month, reserve judgment until the end of the year.
○ Exercise with a friend if possible. Having a workout buddy is a good way to feel "pressured" to continue your fitness regimen. Your friend may need your encouragement as much as you need him or her to urge you on.
○ If you grow bored with your routine, choose a new, equally safe and manageable one.
○ Many people find that buying an exercise video or DVD to use at home helps them stick to working out. There are many selections available, some of which are even geared to those with certain health issues, including MS, and those recovering from injuries. Contact your local chapter of the National Multiple Sclerosis Society (www.nationalmssociety.org) for more information.

○ Stay active while traveling. On business trips, book hotels with health clubs, spas, or pools. Pack your walking sneakers and use them.

IN A SENTENCE:

Whatever your level of fatigue, keep as active as possible, since regular exercise minimizes symptoms and lessens the chance of disability.

Life Choices,
Life Changes

ONCE YOU'VE gotten this far in your first year of living with MS and your treatment is well under way, you may feel a sense of stability once more. As you're coping with the medical realities (and the accompanying uncertainties surrounding this disease), you may wish that everything else in your life would stay the same for a bit. But life doesn't work that way, and nothing stays the same. Even when life isn't presenting new challenges, there are always problems to solve, and things that can work better or be better.

Therefore, now that you've sized up the territory of living with MS, turn your attention to other parts of your life. You may find that there are places where you want to make changes—small ones and big ones. They might be complicated or they might be simple. They could involve physical changes in your environment, such as moving, or emotional changes, such as giving up a relationship gone wrong. Whatever the situation, make your choice of what to do wisely and rationally, and remember that change is very important.

In terms of smaller changes, you may need to make further alterations in your daily routine. Don't be afraid to ask for help.

For example, if you have young children, have your spouse, a friend, or a baby-sitter pick them up from school or at the bus stop.

Similarly, be assertive in speaking up for your own needs. When you are fatigued, make this clear. Lie down and ask your partner, friend, or teenager to go out and get the paper towels and the garbage bags. You will give two important messages: One: I can't do everything. Two: You can definitely help, and I appreciate help when I need it.

Making a move

Sally, a freelance writer, was living in Los Angeles with her husband, Neil, when she was diagnosed with MS. Her major symptoms were fatigue, vision problems, and an unsteady gait. She also did not cope well with heat. She and Neil, a screenwriter, realized quickly that her flare-ups were often triggered by the hot climate of southern California.

The couple spent six uncomfortable months coping with the news of Sally's illness and with some significant flare-ups. For a long time, they had been talking about moving north to Oregon, where they had spent a number of vacations, because the quality of life there seemed better. Now, the added impetus of increasing Sally's chances for good health led them to the decision they had always wanted to make. They soon pulled up stakes and moved to a pleasant home outside Portland. Sally did much of the planning, and Neil did the initial scouting and all of the heavy lifting in order to protect Sally's health.

Needless to say, not everyone has the kind of job flexibility of Sally and Neil, both of whom could work almost anywhere. As described earlier, my friend Carla's "move" was basically from a full-time job as an art director at a food magazine to working freelance. I spoke to Carla recently. She's still working freelance, and she is not only happier, but healthier—she's been doing better, especially regarding fatigue and vision impairment symptoms, since leaving the rat race behind. And she has a new, long-term partner who loves everything about her, including how heroically she manages her symptoms. As she says, "As long as I get to make some decisions for myself, like when I rest and when I eat, I can cope with fatigue and this shaky nerve thing that now and then numbs my right leg." Regardless of what kind of move you make, the lesson from Sally, Neil, and Carla is that the more positive choices and changes you make after your diagnosis, the greater your chances for a happier, less stressful, and healthier future.

Cooling off a difficult relationship

Hannah had a different problem. It involved her mother. Hannah's diagnosis came after a series of bouts with extreme numbness, culminating in near paralysis of her right side. She recovered and began treatment. Over the next month, however, she noticed that each time she spoke to her mother, she began to experience a prolonged period of numbness.

Hannah loves her mother, but knew she had to do something to protect her health. For the rest of her first year living with MS, she chose to speak to her mother only on holidays. "During that time," Hannah reports, "my mom was toxic for me, and guess what? I found the less I told her about everything, the fewer bouts of numbness I had. I was also less upset and had more energy."

Hannah has slowly let her mother back into her life, but at the time she made the right choice for herself. Some people find that parents can be very helpful and supportive, and an adult child who has major problems with symptoms may even physically require a parent's help. No two situations are the same, but if you feel you are managing well on your own, you should not feel guilty about limiting contact with a parent who is overbearing or difficult to cope with in some other way.

The same principle applies with any relative or friend: if a relationship has become difficult, find a way to pull back a bit, so that the stresses don't exacerbate your symptoms.

Calling it quits

Sometimes, withdrawing partially from a difficult relationship isn't enough, as Leslie's story illustrates.

Leslie spent the first six months of her first year trying to work on her relationship with her live-in boyfriend. He had been having reservations whenever they discussed marriage before her diagnosis, so at least she was able to accept that the issues they had to resolve were not caused by her MS status. Finally, she realized the relationship just wasn't going to work— and that her vain efforts to make it work were leaving her exhausted as well as making coping with her MS all the more difficult. Fortunately, he was enough of a gentleman to find another apartment and move out quickly.

The month following her breakup wasn't easy for Leslie, but despite feeling blue and heartsick, she found herself less fatigued. As she came out of the emotional fog that often accompanies ending a serious relationship, she realized she was feeling better than she had since before her diagnosis. Leslie was aware that this was due in large part to the effects of her disease-modifying medication, but she knew that it also had something to do with having made a difficult decision.

For Leslie, making a life change that was emotionally painful was ultimately a good thing—it had helped her to put her health first.

In my case, I was already married when I was diagnosed and couldn't or didn't want to realize how unhappy I was. I had so much on my plate already, what with all my tests, the diagnosis, adjusting to my new status as an MS patient, and learning how to inject myself with Avonex and dealing with the early side effects of the drug. Later, I was able to delve into what wasn't working; for me, it was better that I waited to stabilize my condition and my emotions before tackling another life-changing situation. Remember, it's okay to stay for now, even if the situation isn't great. Just don't feel you have to stay forever. And if this imperfect, maybe even unreliable partner seems like an indispensable crutch to aid you as you limp along to a new sense of balance, you'll realize, as I did once I was on my own again, that your ex was no emotional walking aid, but an impediment to your whole emotional and physical health.

IN A SENTENCE:

> *Making necessary life changes, even disruptive ones, will ultimately help you maintain a positive attitude.*

learning

Complementary and Alternative Medicine

COMPLEMENTARY AND alternative medicine, sometimes abbreviated as CAM, includes everything from chiropractic treatment to aromatherapy. While there was a time
when these kinds of nontraditional treatments were almost
automatically dismissed, these days CAM might even be
termed *accepted* alternative medicine. Almost everyone uses
some form of CAM, even if it's something as minor as drinking
green tea or having a massage. Although the issues that face
those with MS deserve the best of Western medicine, certain
complementary and alternative treatments may be helpful and
will not interfere with the overall treatment.

Caution: I have tried to be evenhanded in my treatment of
these alternative options, but I certainly believe that to discount
disease-modifying treatments is less than likely to be the right
course. On the other hand, I do think that even if the only
result from pursuing an alternative therapy is a "placebo" effect,
this is an area worth exploring. As with any other new item you
want to introduce into your health plan, please consult your
medical team first.

Vitamins and supplements

If you haven't noticed already, a visit to a pharmacy, a health-food store, or a vitamin boutique will convince you that we live in a culture of "the pill." The aisles are stocked with hundreds of choices, from pills for illnesses and pain relief to vitamin and supplement tablets. The bottles entice with all kinds of benefits: they cure various ills and alleviate the symptoms of others; they enhance athletic, mental, and sexual performance; they increase energy levels; and so on. And it doesn't stop there. We've also been inundated with a tempting array of tinctures, extracts, and oils that also promise to help us reach the promised land of perfect health.

All these promises can be awfully tempting, particularly when you are faced with the mystery of MS. If you want to augment your treatment with vitamin therapy, there are some supplements commonly recommended for treatment of MS that you should know about. For additional information, you may want to consult a nutritionist. In any event, proceed cautiously and carefully. Consult your MS specialist before taking any new vitamins, minerals, or other supplements. If you have already regularly been taking a multiple vitamin, make sure you mention it.

Antioxidants. Antioxidants neutralize free radicals, chemicals that can damage cells in organs of the body, including the brain. Vitamins A, C, and E are the most common antioxidants.

While antioxidants are a popular supplement, for those with MS, the situation is more complicated. As with so many other things, there are pros and cons for you to consider before you take these vitamins.

On the one hand, evidence shows that antioxidants may work to minimize the damage caused to nerve cells in MS. Immune cells called *macrophages* release these free radicals, which not only cause injury to the myelin sheath covering your nerve cells but can also damage the axon, or body of the cell. This would indicate that people with MS would benefit from taking more antioxidants.

However, antioxidants do not affect macrophage cells only. They also are thought to boost immune-system function. This might affect the immune system, which is already too active in those of us with MS.

Before you tie yourself up in knots deciding what to do, keep in mind that antioxidants are already present in many of the nutritious foods you eat, and no one has told you to stop eating . . . yet. It's best to discuss the matter with your doctor. If you and your doctor decide it's okay for you to take an antioxidant supplement, try the lowest doses of vitamins A, C, and E. It is unlikely that moderate amounts of these vitamins will cause any further stimulation to your immune system, and such doses may help your body neutralize free radicals with less damage to presently healthy cells. If you take only one of these vitamins, try vitamin C, which might help you fend off colds that could exacerbate symptoms.

One other antioxidant you should know about is Coenzyme Q10 (CoQ10). It has been found to be helpful in treating certain heart conditions, probably because it improves the function of mitochondria, the energy-producing components of the body's cells. This can be particularly important in maintaining healthy blood flow, which may be helpful in issues involving circulation for someone with MS. Once again, proceed with caution and, if you do decide to take CoQ10, start with a low dose.

The vitamin Bs. For years some experts and many nonexperts have thought that a deficiency of vitamin B_{12} played a role in the development of MS. But studies of vitamin B_{12} deficiencies in those with MS have produced inconclusive results, and there is no evidence that B_{12} deficiency causes neurological impairment.

A reasonable dosage of all the B vitamins (including folic acid or folate) is included in any recommended daily vitamin, and supplementary dosages should not be taken. In particular, vitamins B_6 (pyridoxine) and B_3 (niacin) should be avoided in large doses. More than 50 milligrams a day of B_6 has been associated with nerve damage. More than 35 milligrams a day of B_3 can injure the liver, raise blood-sugar levels, and cause flushing and nausea.

Milk thistle. Numerous controlled studies in Germany have demonstrated that milk thistle can aid the liver in returning to health. Why should you worry about your liver if you have MS? Avonex, Copaxone, and most of the other injectable treatments tax your liver. Antibiotics may also tax your liver, as can the chronic use of medications like ibuprofen and Imodium A-D.

In terms of protecting your liver, it's hard to find anything bad to say about milk thistle. The medical debate regarding the claims for milk thistle continues, but there is a growing consensus that it does aid in the regeneration of the surface cells of the liver, and there is an ever-increasing barrage of patient testimony to its positive effects. It is an accepted addition to protocols in Europe for medical treatment and a supplement widely used by Americans who want to take more part in their own medical care. There are various capsules available in this country, such as the Nature's Way brand, Thisilyn-Maximum Absorption Formula. It is also agreed that milk thistle is an invaluable aid in many skin conditions, including acne, and as an aid in increasing general skin tone and vitality. Since the side effects are minimal to nonexistent, it's a good bet for your health regimen. Both my son and I take it, and I can say without a doubt that his acne flare-ups happen with less frequency and that many people remark on how great (and wrinkle free) my skin looks.

Acidophilus and biphodopholous. The body needs "good bacterias" like acidophilus and biphodopholous to stay healthy. If you can afford a supplement that includes acidophilus and biphodopholous, take it. This supplement may also help women manage vaginal infections.

Evening primrose oil. Although there is still debate in the medical community over whether or not evening primrose oil can help reduce inflammation and the recurrence of episodes in those coping with MS, the overall picture for this oil as a health aid in many illnesses and conditions (arthritis, PMS, and eczema, to name a few) looks good. New studies have shown that the oil helps to lower your level of LDL (bad) cholesterol. Evening primrose oil, sold in capsules or caplets, is rich in the essential fatty acid gamma-linolenic acid (GLA). Some researchers claim that people with MS have a deficiency of GLA in their systems. GLA helps the body produce prostaglandins, which increase blood flow as well as reduce inflammation and blood clotting. If your doctor does give the okay for you to try the oil, begin with a minimal dosage and monitor how your system reacts.

Ginkgo biloba extract. Ginkgo biloba extract (GBE), from the leaves of the ginkgo biloba tree, is being recommended for the treatment of cognitive dysfunction in the aging population and for those dealing with MS in particular. Research has shown that ginkgo biloba extract can neutralize the toxins released by the white blood cells in the brain and thus limit memory loss and other aspects of cognitive dysfunction. Clinical trials are currently under way to see how effective ginkgo biloba extract actually is.

Acupuncture

Acupuncture, a major component of traditional Chinese medicine, is based on the theory that free-flowing energy, called "qi" (or chi), travels along fourteen meridians in the body. In acupuncture, a special type of needle is inserted just under the skin at the "acupoints" along these meridians in order to correct, rebalance, and stimulate energy flow. Believers say that such treatments can relieve pain and treat many health problems, including asthma, addiction, ulcers, and the common cold. However, the jury is still out on how acupuncture affects the immune system. Studies offer conflicting information, ranging from claims that acupuncture activates the immune system to claims that it inhibits the immune system.

If you used acupuncture before your diagnosis and found it helpful to your overall health, you should discuss whether you should continue to use it with your doctor. He or she may suggest a hiatus from the treatment until you have started your treatment regimen and your condition has been stabilized.

Homeopathy

Homeopathy is based on the idea that "like treats like." For example, since large doses of arsenic cause stomach cramps and intestinal disorders, homeopathic principles say that very small doses of arsenic would then be successful in treating severe stomach cramps.

The merits of homeopathy remain a matter of much debate among professionals, and there have been no rigorous studies to determine homeopathy's effectiveness in treating MS. If you are oriented toward alternative therapies, you may want to consider homeopathy for mild conditions, such as low-level pain, a viral infection, or minor anxiety. But always check with your doctor first. In general, homeopathy is considered a low-risk therapy. The costs tend to be moderate and affordable, unless a person becomes obsessed with homeopathic products. In most cases, the success of homeopathic treatments seems to be related to their ability to draw on the placebo effect—a person *thinks* he or she feels better, therefore the person *does feel* better.

Chiropractic medicine

These days, chiropractic medicine is one of the most accepted forms of CAM, having come a long way from the years when the American Medical Association disparaged and discredited it. Many insurance companies now cover at least a portion of chiropractic treatment, as do Medicare and

Medicaid. Every year, more than 15 million Americans use the services of a chiropractor and come away satisfied. And many people attest to chiropractic medicine contributing to their overall sense of "wellness."

It's also the largest field of CAM in the United States: chiropractors are the third largest group of health-care practitioners, after medical doctors and dentists. Chiropractors tend to do a responsible, professional job in managing a patient's pain, and most respectable chiropractors know when to say that something is beyond their jurisdiction as a health professional. My own chiropractor referred another of his patients, a woman in her thirties, to a neurologist, and she was diagnosed with MS and is receiving treatment.

The basic idea underlying chiropractic medicine is that slight abnormalities of the spine may be responsible for medical problems affecting other portions of the body. These musculoskeletal abnormalities are fixed by correcting the alignment of the spine, usually by manipulation. While there are few studies regarding chiropractic treatment of MS symptoms, common sense suggests that by keeping your spine aligned correctly, you may be able to help yourself with balance and gait, as well as stiffness and spasticity. What studies have shown clearly is that people with MS suffering from short-term lower back pain do benefit from chiropractic treatment.

Spinal manipulation is only part of modern chiropractic practice. Chiropractors are also schooled in working on other parts of the body. For example, my chiropractor worked on the scar tissue that resulted from the fall down stairs that I mentioned earlier, which itself led to my MS diagnosis.

Chiropractors increasingly use ultrasound therapy as well. If issues of balance have affected your gait, for instance, and this in turn has started to bother you, treating the affected area with ultrasound helps relieve pain, allowing you to begin fixing any bad walking habits you adopted to compensate for the discomfort.

Once again, speak to your MS specialist or internist before going forward with chiropractic treatment, especially if you have other conditions, such as hypertension.

Massage

Therapeutic massage by a licensed massage therapist is good for you in general, whatever your health issues may be. It can relieve symptoms of MS, such as spasticity, numbness, and even tremor. In fact, studies have shown that therapeutic massage plays a part in reducing fatigue, anxiety, stress, and even depression, all of which exacerbate symptoms of MS.

The relaxation and increased circulation that massage induces are both beneficial to anyone coping with MS and to feelings of well-being in general. Massage may also do a great deal for your self-esteem. Called "the loving touch," massage tends to make you feel closer to your physical self. Many people report it's a liberating relief to have a caring professional work on their limbs and muscles.

Before the session begins, tell your massage therapist about any recent injuries, since those areas should not be massaged. The therapist generally leaves the room while you undress and cover yourself with a sheet, towel, or blanket. Your massage therapist will either work through the covering or expose only the body part that is being treated. If you don't want your body to be exposed at all, tell your massage therapist beforehand. Also speak up if you feel too warm or too cold during the massage.

Reflexology

Reflexology therapy is based on the theory that applying pressure to specific areas on the bottom of the foot will affect wellness in different parts of the body—each area of the sole is supposedly a reflex point for a corresponding area of the body. The intention of reflexology is to increase energy flow to the specific area of the body that is giving you trouble and, therefore, improve health.

While studies on the efficacy of reflexology in the treatment of disease are limited, it is painless and relaxing and, like massage therapy, it may have emotional benefits. Some people with MS have reported that reflexology helps manage their fatigue.

The water the feet are bathed in is cool, a good start for those of us with MS who are heat sensitive, and the tenor of the foot massage is one of calm and relaxation. Sessions usually last thirty or sixty minutes, and the cost is reasonable. If you have the time, the financial resources, and the inclination, reflexology can be a way of stimulating energy and resting the mind. If nothing else, it is also a pleasant way of paying special attention to your feet.

Other therapies

There are a few other alternative therapies that have their advocates in the MS community. While the merits of these treatments are a matter of ongoing debate, it's worth taking a brief look at them. For one thing, you are your own person and you need to make your own choices. If an alternative therapy intrigues you, get more information about it (see Resources) and discuss it with your doctor.

In addition, even if skeptics say these therapies have no physical benefit, they may make you feel better. As you know, there is a connection between stress levels, how you manage the stress you do have, and your MS. People who maintain a positive attitude have a better chance of managing life's stresses successfully. Few things put a damper on a positive attitude more quickly than a sense of hopelessness and being out of control. If any of these therapies contributes to your sense of well-being and of control, you will feel better, and that in turn will keep your stress levels down.

Hippotherapy. No, we're not talking about hippopotamuses, but hippotherapy shares the same Greek root, *hippos*, meaning "horse." As the name suggests, it's the use of horseback riding as therapy. Dating back to Greece in the fifth century B.C.E., riding therapy came into vogue in Europe in the twentieth century. It is now catching on in the United States, with more than six hundred accredited therapeutic riding centers.

In regard to MS, the theory behind hippotherapy is that following the motions of the horse improves a problematic gait and can strengthen weakened leg muscles. Riding is supposed to help improve walking for those who are experiencing walking unsteadiness, because the rhythmic motion of the human pelvis while riding emulates the movement of the pelvis while walking. Studies are currently under way to test the merits of hippotherapy in treating those with MS, cerebral palsy, or other diseases of the CNS.

Of course, there is the possible side effect of falling off the horse, which, while something anyone could do without, is particularly dangerous to the MS patient. Falls can cause a relapse or an exacerbation. For safety reasons, therefore, you should ride only at a stable accredited for hippotherapy. In addition, you should discuss your adventure in riding with your specialist before ever getting on a horse.

Hyperbaric oxygen therapy. In hyperbaric oxygen therapy (HBOT), you are placed inside an oxygen chamber. The atmospheric pressure in the chamber is then elevated, the goal being to introduce greater amounts of oxygen into the body's tissues. (Whether this actually occurs is the question asked by doubting Thomases.)

Supporters of HBOT insist that it does oxygenate the blood and enhances the immune system. Some practitioners also claim that HBOT facilitates the production of myelin and helps minimize symptoms of MS, including bladder and bowel dysfunction. Some people swear by HBOT and others categorize it as one more fad. As yet, none of the claims made by advocates of HBOT and MS treatment have been proven.

Bovine myelin. Advocates of bovine myelin therapy believe that the underlying and unequivocal cause of MS is an ongoing autoimmune attack on the myelin sheaths in the CNS. They also believe that the myelin found in cows is similar enough to the myelin found in humans that it can be used interchangeably. The idea behind this highly experimental treatment is that consuming bovine myelin capsules will help to desensitize the immune system, thereby blunting autoimmune reactions.

The effectiveness of this treatment is yet to be proven.

Bee venom treatment. Bee venom treatment (BVT) is last on the list because it is more controversial and more expensive than any of the others discussed. In addition, it can be very risky and may cause severe, even life-threatening side effects and complications. While there are those who swear that it has improved their condition, they tend to be people with relapsing-remitting MS whose condition would have improved anyway.

Advocates of this treatment claim that repeated injections of poisonous bee venom impact the immune system in ways that may suppress symptoms of MS and even reverse the condition. The venom used is from the common honeybee (*Apis mellifera*). In the quantities used in these injections, the treatment can be dangerous and even lethal.

If you are having enough trouble simply trying to adjust to a daily or weekly injection of a fully tested and safe medication for the treatment of MS, BVT is definitely not for you. On the other hand, if you are the type that enjoys a certain amount of medical bungee jumping, you may want to look into the therapy. Information on BVT is available through the American Apitherapy Society, or ASS. (Apis is the Greek word for bee.) Those who are on a beta-blocker cannot use BVT, nor can anyone with a history of anaphylactic reactions or who has experienced anaphylactic shock. As with any other controversial alternative therapy for MS, consult with your physician.

IN A SENTENCE:

> *Some people with MS report benefits from taking vitamin supplements or pursuing alternative medicine, but consult your medical team first.*

Traveling with MS

AS YOU'VE dealt with your diagnosis over the past five months, begun to get treatment, and made the necessary adjustments in many areas of your life, you probably have stayed closer to home than in the past. However, having MS does not restrict you to your hometown and the surrounding area. Now that you have come this far, you can and should think about returning to your normal travel schedule, whether it is for business or pleasure.

Planning a trip

Traveling, particularly air travel, has changed a lot since September 11, 2001. Long delays are common. Everything from knitting needles to nail clippers may be considered potential weapons. Prepare for delays, and if you haven't traveled in a while, ask other travelers what you might expect. Make sure you carry photo I.D., such as a driver's license or passport. Try to take your medication at the same time each day while traveling as you do when you are at home, and whether you inject once a week or three days a week, try to stick to the same schedule on the road.

Regardless of how often you inject yourself, before traveling get a letter from your MS specialist confirming that you manage MS by self-injecting medication. The best thing to do is to get a general letter that you can use over and over for ordinary vacations and domestic trips. This letter can also be helpful in case of delays or other problems en route and in case you need special services in an overcrowded terminal.

Bring the phone numbers of your doctors, just in case. If you are going on a long trip, have been experiencing symptoms, or have just recovered from a relapse, ask your doctor if he or she can recommend a doctor or hospital near your destination and bring that number with you.

For international destinations or a longer trip, you might want a more detailed letter, plus duplicate prescriptions for antibiotics and painkillers, just in case.

When you travel overseas, make a photocopy of the first spread of your passport; pack it, together with spare passport photographs, in a separate location from the passport in case your important documents are lost or stolen.

If you will be giving yourself your shots while you are away, call your hotel and make sure that a refrigerator will be available to you in order to store your medication. For longer trips, also inquire whether your hotel has laundry and dry-cleaning facilities, so you can pack less clothing.

As you prepare to pack, remember to travel light. Use travel-size containers of cosmetics, tissues, and anything else you can think of. For a longer trip, consider shipping anything heavy, such as books, to your destination by UPS or another package courier.

If you're going on a long trip, here's a tip from Bill, the man who has trouble walking but can ride a bicycle perfectly. He had always groused about how he could get only four doses of medicine at one time, covering just a month. But as he made arrangements to spend six weeks in India, he was thrilled (and mollified) to learn that the company that manufactured the medication would indeed use a courier service to send his dosage overseas. Federal Express delivered Bill's medicine on time and to the right address in India.

As you pack, keep your meds and a sharps container (for used needles) in your carry-on luggage.

If you don't already have luggage with built-in wheels, invest in such bags now. Even if you are almost symptom-free, you will want to avoid carrying luggage whenever possible.

Dealing with Extended Travel

IF YOU are going to be away for some time, you may want to get your itinerary in place early on and ask your insurance carrier's pharmacy connection to airmail the medications to your destination. If you are traveling for two months or more, this could mean two or three new addresses. Most carriers are well equipped to do this. It will save you all sorts of complications in terms of getting through security and, most important, ensuring the refrigeration, and therefore the potency and safety of your medication. (Keep in mind that the more you make friends with your insurance carrier and all connected resources, the more likely you are to get as close to what you need from them.)

Business travel

When it comes to business travel, corporations look to get the most bang for their buck. If you have already traveled on business, you are probably aware of how these trips can be tightly scheduled with an unspoken agenda to go, go, go.

In arranging your first business trip after your diagnosis, discuss the itinerary and schedule with your boss. After assuring him or her that you are in good shape and look forward to accomplishing the goals of the trip, make sure it's clear that you need a more relaxed schedule than normal. You want to reserve your strength for the important things and not to overload your days. Try to schedule adequate rest time. For instance, skip the business dinner after a long day on site at a client's (if you know the client well, you can explain why you need your rest; for others, it's enough to say that unfortunately you are unavailable for dinner).

The Ever-Shifting Rules for Flying

THE NEWEST restrictions on how we travel by air, imposed in the summer of 2006, restrict the amount of liquids and gels in the cabin. Fortunately, this will hardly affect those of us who cope with MS at all—except, of course, in terms of waiting time.

It is the same deal as with your syringes. Bring your prescription and a letter from your doctor, and you will be allowed to take your medication on board with you.

If you're taking Avonex, your trip is short, and you are well established in your medication regimen, you might think of injecting yourself at home, a day early before departure or a day late after return, in order to avoid taking syringes. With Copaxone, which is injected daily, and Rebif, which is injected three times a week, you'll need to bring your syringes with you.

Although rules for flying keep changing, as long as you're well prepared, you will always be able to keep your medications with you. Do not worry.

Travel by air

Given that you may be adjusting to a disease-modifying medication regimen, and you really don't need the jet lag right now, it makes sense to consider limiting your air travel for the first year after your diagnosis. Of course, you may well find yourself in a situation (for instance, for your job) that requires you to fly. There are a few things you can do to make air travel a bit easier.

The first commandment of traveling successfully is to carry all your medications with you on board the plane. This may be more difficult with the present security restrictions, but your doctor's letter will ease the way for you. Because your medication and the needles you use are tightly packaged, you should be able to manage to keep your medication with you, although keep in mind that every airport and each screening may present a new obstacle.

Carry your oral meds in your purse, briefcase, or other carry-on bag. Use a small, insulated lunch bag to hold your Avonex, Copaxone, or other MS medication. To be extra careful about keeping your Avonex cool, put a small ice pack in the bag with the medication.

If you are taking a flight with meal service, you can call the airline up to forty-eight hours before your flight to order a special meal (e.g., low-fat or kosher). Now that in-flight meal service is rarer, some travelers prepare their own meal at home or buy something nutritious at the terminal, carry it on board, and eat it aloft.

You may also want to inquire about services available at the airport, such as curbside check-in, or a porter to carry your luggage for you. If you do need assistance, call ahead to make the necessary arrangements.

Airborne Advice

○ As usual, drink plenty of water, but make sure you've got your sights on a bathroom—in the airport, on the plane, and at your destination. (Although this goes without saying, sometimes we need to be reminded!)

○ Reserve a seat on the aisle; this will give you easier access to the lavatory and also help you get off the plane more quickly.

○ If the flight is providing meal service, reserve a special meal beforehand.

○ To keep from dealing with unnecessary searches, make sure you carry a letter in your wallet from your doctor stating that you have MS and must inject yourself for your therapy. Bring something for your sharps, such as a small Tupperware container.

○ Use a suitcase on rollers and don't overpack. Even if you still feel in complete control, you don't want to tax yourself more than you have to.

○ If you already have some mobility issues, ask to board first. You deserve the privilege. (And use the bathroom at the gate before you board.)

○ If you want to stay hydrated but you don't want to walk to the bathroom all that often, remember you can also hydrate from the outside. Facial sprays (such as Evian or one of the organic sprays with an herbal base) can be found at your local health-food store. If it's allowed, carry one when you fly, spraying you face every now and then to moisturize and soothe.

○ If you suffer from fatigue, or if you have experienced an exacerbation lately and feel you need a little support—emotionally or physically—arrange to have a friend or family member or a business associate meet you at the airport when you arrive.

Travel by train

If you are traveling a short distance, the train can be a convenient alternative to air travel, particularly in the Northeast. The Acela Express trains running from Washington, D.C., to Boston can be faster door to door than flying, especially on shorter segments of the trip, such as Philadelphia to New York City. You don't have to get to the train station far in advance and you avoid the wear and tear of getting to and from the airport.

When you travel by train, you will not have to go through security checkpoints. While a letter from your doctor is therefore not as important, it's still a good idea to carry one with you. You will also be able to keep your luggage with you, thereby avoiding hassles about lost luggage and being able to keep your medication with you.

Travel by car

Traveling by car can be grueling, especially on a long drive. However, it has many advantages, including letting you pack exactly what you want to pack, putting the things you will need during the day in the car and the rest in the trunk. You can carry a cooler filled with sandwiches, snacks, and cold drinks, as well as a second, smaller cooler for your medication. If you are traveling with your children, you can bring games to keep them amused. You can alter your route at the spur of the moment, taking detours to see interesting sights or pulling into a rest stop when you need to relax.

Prepare for a road trip by mapping your route and studying it beforehand. Put a flashlight and a magnifying glass in the glove compartment, to help you read the map after dark. If you are traveling with another adult, discuss how to split up the driving. If your companion does it all, consider yourself lucky and keep your favorite pillow in the backseat, so you can nap when desired.

On longer road trips, monitor whether you're getting fatigued. Don't hesitate to stop at a motel along the route if you just can't make your destination in one day.

Once again, you'll want to bring the phone numbers of your doctors with you, and copies of any prescriptions you might need filled while away.

At your destination

At your hotel, make sure your room is located close to fire exits. If you have any problems with mobility, a room closer to elevators or on a lower floor is a good bet. Don't be shy about asking to change your room.

As you get settled into your home away from home, choose a table with enough light and make this your designated injection area. Always put your sharps container back in your suitcase so you don't leave it in your hotel room by mistake.

IN A SENTENCE:

Careful planning will make traveling with MS easy.

learning

The Ins and Outs of Insurance

HEALTH INSURANCE seems to be in a continual state of crisis in the United States, with new systems being introduced, government pressure to keep costs down, the new Medicare Part D that provides prescription coverage for senior citizens, and the continuing problem of the uninsured. Many people don't have to fully understand the ins and outs of their insurance coverage, but anyone with a chronic condition such as MS doesn't have that luxury. You'll need to learn as much as possible about your plan so that you get all the benefits to which you are entitled.

The uninsured

Sara had symptoms of MS in her early thirties but was not officially diagnosed until she was forty-two. Six years later, she still has no health insurance. "But that's okay," she says. "I tell myself that I have to stay healthy, and it helps motivate me."

It is a tribute to Sara that she can be so calm, wise, and even positive about this situation. Nevertheless, it is a sad state of affairs that, according to U.S. Bureau of the Census statistics for the year 2004, 45.8 million Americans had no form of health-insurance coverage. The poor, the foreign-born, people of color, and young adults are more likely to be uninsured.

A recent study by the Institute of Medicine at The National Academies reports that the uninsured become ill more often than those with insurance, and they also die earlier. This finding is predictable—facing an optional and expensive screening examination or early detection tests for a chronic condition such as MS, cancer, diabetes, and the like, many uninsured pass on the procedure, and then don't get diagnosed until they're sicker—but it's still alarming.

If you have any choice in the matter, don't let yourself become one of the uninsured. That said, we must all work in our own small ways to change the system so that insurance for all becomes a possibility and not just a dream.

Navigating the insurance maze

Even if you are insured, it can be frustratingly difficult to cope with the system at the same time that you are just learning to cope with MS. The system is full of all kinds of hurdles that you have to jump to get the benefits your insurance company has promised you in its policy.

One of the biggest hurdles is access to the facts of what's covered and at what percentage of reimbursement. Many private insurance companies or managed-care plans don't make it easy for you to get the information you need to know. In general, insurance woes have increased for everyone; however, in terms of coverage for the established and the newer disease-modifying therapies, the news is actually improving. Many of the larger health insurance companies, including Aetna and Empire Blue Cross, do cover most of these therapies and even provide pharmaceutical services and delivery of your medication for only a small co-pay. For example, Aetna uses the pharmaceutical services of Avonex-Direct; Empire Blue Cross uses Care-Marc. These companies deliver the medication on a monthly basis and even call you at the end of each month to recheck your order and all essential information, and answer any further questions you might have. I have found their performance to be exemplary and their care and attentiveness to be indispensable. I spoke to Care-Marc regarding coverage of Tysabri once it becomes available, and that, too, will be covered. Two federal laws, the Consolidated Omnibus Budget Reconciliation Act (COBRA) and the Health Insurance Portability and Accountability Act (HIPAA), ensure that if you are covered by a group health plan, you can maintain your coverage and guarantee your future insurability.

The website of the National Multiple Sclerosis Society (NMSS) is one of the best in terms of offering you concrete information on insurance companies. However, be leery of any websites sponsored by insurance companies—the information there may not be unbiased.

Additionally, NMSS now has a short book available that helps people with MS navigate the various complexities of insurance coverage. You can contact your local chapter of the society to obtain a copy, or order it on the website.

According to the NMSS, even if someone with MS does have insurance coverage, in most cases the coverage is inadequate for the person's needs. In informal surveys by the NMSS, the most often noted areas where needs were left unmet are:

- O Medication coverage
- O Rehabilitation-services coverage, especially physical therapy
- O Reimbursement for necessary medical equipment
- O Home-care coverage

These unmet needs are often attributed to the refusal of many health-insurance companies to sell initial coverage to, or continue coverage with, a person with a so-called *preexisting condition*. A preexisting condition refers to any mental or physical condition for which you obtained treatment within the six months before your enrollment in an insurance plan, and the plans are written to exclude coverage of such conditions. Sydney Lewis, author of *Hospital*, jokes, "Insurance companies seem to consider birth a preexisting condition," but it's no laughing matter if you are already diagnosed with MS and you have to switch insurance carriers because of a change in your job or your personal status. Insurance companies have also been known to restrict coverage for people with a preexisting condition or disability.

The NMSS and other like-minded organizations are dedicated to helping those with MS navigate the labyrinthine world of insurance and to finding ways to improve the current insurance system.

The NMSS has published "Accessing the Disease-Modifying Drugs for the Newly Diagnosed." Call or write the NMSS national office to obtain this excellent free brochure about getting your disease-modifying therapy and to locate the NMSS chapter in your area (see Resources).

A Note About Coverage

NEEDLESS TO say, everyone with MS deserves medical insurance coverage in order to receive the care they need. While this is not yet the case, progress is being made, particularly in terms of reimbursement for the expensive disease-modifying medications. If you are having problems with your existing coverage or are simply trying to obtain coverage, discuss the situation with your doctor. He or she and the staff have the most firsthand experience with the insurance companies. When you have questions about your insurance options, call your local NMSS chapter and ask for information—they are always willing to help.

Types of insurance coverage

Before you were diagnosed with MS, you may never have had to focus on the kind of insurance plan you have. Perhaps the coverage comes through your spouse's job, and he or she has always dealt with the paperwork. Or maybe, because your plan routinely handled claims for simple checkups and medical situations, it never seemed that problematic. Now that things have changed, and you have more doctors' visits, more medications to take, and special needs, you may need to learn more about the different types of coverage that are available.

Here is a brief overview of the present options.

FEE-FOR-SERVICE PLANS

This is the kind of medical insurance that most of us grew up with, and some people still have such a plan. Over the last quarter century, however, fee-for-service plans have been increasingly replaced by managed-care plans, such as HMOs and PPOs. Bills are submitted to the insurance company and, after you meet an annual deductible, the insurance company pays a portion of the fee (usually 50 to 80 percent) and you pay the rest.

The advantage of a fee-for-service plan is that typically you can see any doctor you want, without a referral. However, these plans are much rarer in the twenty-first century and if you can get one, it's expensive. Your employer may ask for a hefty contribution toward the cost of a fee-for-service policy, and you are responsible for the portion of the fees the insurance company does not cover. With MS, this could add up.

Health maintenance organizations (HMOs)

The oldest type of managed-care plans, HMOs spread across the country in the 1980s and 1990s. Basically, this is a prepaid insurance plan that provides agreed-upon services for a standard premium. The HMO has a network of associated doctors and other health-care professionals, all of whom have agreed to accept set fees in return for a minimum of paperwork. This group of physicians and others is referred to as the *network*. A doctor who is not associated with your particular HMO is said to be *out of network*.

When you enroll in an HMO, you must designate one doctor, usually an internist, as your primary-care physician. That doctor acts as the central provider of your health care. You cannot go to a specialist of any kind without a referral slip from your primary-care physician. (If you do, the HMO will not cover the visit, even if the specialist is in the network.)

The HMO encourages you to stay within its network. Most HMOs require a small *co-pay*, or fixed amount, for each office visit with an in-network doctor. Whenever you go out of network, the financial burdens shift to you, the patient. Coverage of visits to any out-of-network professional is limited at best—usually, you alone are responsible for the charges.

Generally, the HMO must be informed, via a toll-free number, before any hospitalization.

An HMO can work fine as long as all members of your medical team are in the network. Premiums are generally lower than with preferred-provider organizations (PPOs), the other principal kind of managed-care plan in the United States.

Preferred-provider organizations (PPOs)

As consumers and health-care advocates expressed concerns about the restrictions of HMOs, a newer kind of managed-care plan became popular in the last decade. A preferred-provider organization (PPO) offers economic incentives to see its doctors, but it is more flexible than an HMO.

A PPO also sets up a network of doctors who contract with it and receive set fees in exchange for less paperwork. However, you do not need a referral from your primary-care physician to see a specialist. If you go to a specialist who is not in the PPO's network, the PPO provides limited coverage: you will be asked to meet an annual deductible, and you will be responsible for covering the most costly charges for treatment or to share significantly in these costs.

When you stay in its network, the co-pay for a doctor's visit is slightly higher in a PPO than in an HMO. Again, hospital stays must be authorized in advance.

MEDICARE AND MEDICAID

Available to almost all Americans sixty-five or older, Medicare is a federal health-insurance program. It is also open to those who have qualified for disability checks through the Social Security program. Although Medicare has encouraged its users to enroll in HMOs and PPOs, most people choose the basic program, a fee-for-service plan. Premiums are deducted monthly from your Social Security check. Under the fee-for-service plan, there is a $110 deductible per year, which you must pay; after that, Medicare pays 80 percent of most doctors' visits and procedures, and you are responsible for the rest. The Medicare Part D program inaugurated in 2006 provides many elderly Americans with prescription-drug coverage. Many senior citizens purchase so-called supplementary insurance, to help with the portion of health-care costs that Medicare doesn't pay for, and to cover the high costs of many drugs.

Medicaid is intended for those on public assistance and the very poor. Sometimes a person of modest means on Medicare with chronic health problems will exhaust his or her personal resources; at that point, it's possible to qualify for Medicaid.

To learn more and find out whether you qualify for either program, talk to a social worker or contact your local Social Security office or your chapter of the NMSS.

Getting Help with Insurance Issues

THERE IS no such thing as great health insurance, but there are ways to improve your options. If you need to fight back, here are some resources:

Consumer Coalition for Quality Health Care
1275 K Street NW, Suite 602
Washington, DC 20005
202–789–3606
www.consumers.org

Center for Patient Advocacy
1350 Beverly Road, Suite 108
McLean, VA 22101
800–846–7444 or 703–748–0400
www.patientadvocacy.org.

Consumers for Quality Care
1750 Ocean Park Avenue, Suite 200
Santa Monica, CA 90405
310–392–0522
www.consumerwatchdog.org

You might also want to contact the Council for Affordable Health Insurance (www.cahi.org/index.asp). This national organization provides not only information on the issues, but also publications, resources, consumer information, and upcoming seminars and events.

Additionally, William M. Shernoff's *Fight Back and Win: How to Get Your HMO and Health Insurance to Pay Up* is an excellent guide to getting your HMO to do what it's supposed to. You can find this book at your local bookshop or at any online retailer.

Getting the most out of your insurance plan

Knowing what kind of coverage you have doesn't answer the next important question: Will your plan cover the medication of your choice, and to what extent? This can be a problem if a medication or therapy has recently been introduced, since insurance companies can be slow to accept new medical options as valid, and may refuse to reimburse them.

To find out how much coverage you have, consult the benefits administrator at your company regarding your coverage. Otherwise, you can call the insurance carrier directly. Write down your concerns ahead of time, so you make sure you get all the information you need. Here are some important questions:

○ Will you need to review my case before my therapy is approved?
○ Will I need a letter from my specialist accompanying any prescription order?
○ What percentage of my therapy will be covered?
○ Is there a yearly or lifetime cap on my coverage?

If you have trouble getting the answers you need, an organization named MSActiveSource may be able to help you. As a patient using Avonex, I found their reimbursement counselors extremely helpful. See the Resource list at the back of the book.

An excellent source for information on managing insurance issues when you have a chronic disease is Laura Cooper's book *Insurance Solutions— Plan Well, Live Better: A Workbook for People with a Chronic Disease or Disability* (see For Further Reading).

Save all records and receipts in labeled folders in a safe and convenient location. If you tend to forget where you put papers or if you tend to misplace things, ask for a second copy of every bill at the doctor's office or make one yourself, and keep a duplicate file.

One good thing about many HMOs and PPOs is that as long as you stay in network, you yourself don't have to file claims or do a lot of paperwork. However, if you have a plan where you yourself need to file claims, consider batching your submissions. You can go crazy between the paperwork and keeping track of reimbursements if you file a claim after each doctor's visit.

If your finances allow, wait until you have enough charges that add up to a substantial reimbursement check. This is one of the reasons to be conscientious about all medical receipts.

If you have been billed for a major test and money is tight, it is okay to ignore the first bill and pay the second one (this is a case, however, where you want to submit your claim right away, without waiting for others to make a batch). If you have a credit card, use it whenever possible to pay for a doctor's visit. This means you can file for reimbursement (using your doctor's receipt as proof of the visit) without really paying for the visit until your credit card bill comes due. This is what buying time is all about.

To avoid becoming overwhelmed as you file claims, track whether you or your doctor have been reimbursed (and to the proper amount), and follow up on the problems that invariably occur when dealing with insurance companies. Get help. Help may mean anything from inviting a friend over to give you moral support as you fill out the claim forms to hiring a bookkeeper. If your immediate reaction to the latter suggestion is that it would be too expensive, think creatively. You may have a friend or acquaintance who keeps the books for a small business such as a restaurant and who may be able to assist you a few hours each month, for a nominal fee.

IN A SENTENCE:

> *Learn all you can about your insurance coverage, so that you will have access to the treatment and therapy you need and get reimbursed properly.*

HALF-YEAR MILESTONE

Now that you are halfway through your first year with multiple sclerosis, you have:

○ ACCEPTED THE IDEA THAT MS WILL BE PART OF YOUR LIFE FOREVER.

○ LEARNED TO TAKE CARE OF YOURSELF TO THE BEST OF YOUR ABILITY, BUT WHEN YOU NEED HELP, YOU ASK FOR IT.

○ TAKEN CHARGE OF YOUR HEALTH AND ACCEPTED THE IMPORTANCE OF A HEALTHY DIET AND EXERCISE REGIMEN.

○ RECOGNIZED THAT THIS IS A DISEASE THAT CANNOT DEFEAT YOU. YOUR LEGITI-MATE ANGER WON'T DEFEAT YOUR PUR-POSE, WHICH IS TO BE AS PRODUCTIVE, POSITIVE, AND ABLE AS POSSIBLE IN ALL ASPECTS OF LIFE. YOU HAVE NOT ALLOWED MS TO BE THE FOCUS OF YOUR LIFE—IT IS SIMPLY ANOTHER ASPECT OF YOUR LIFE, WHICH YOU DEAL WITH AS WELL AS YOU CAN.

○ Maintained a positive attitude and self-image, even if you have symptoms or a relapse.

○ Not allowed fear to interfere with your progress. You have taken charge and are looking forward to your future.

Home Safety for MS

YOUR HOME should be a refuge for you, a place of comfort where you can relax in a secure, safe environment. Those of us with MS have special needs that may necessitate some changes being made to our home environment. Most important, with balance issues a major component of the disease, we have to be alert about situations that could lead a person to fall.

Avoiding falls at home

While falling down isn't good for anyone, it is much more perilous for a person with MS who is experiencing symptoms, having a relapse, or is already partially disabled. Here are some quick fixes that be can done at little expense to help prevent falls.

- Use rubber, nonskid matting under any runners, small rugs, or throw rugs. You may want to consider dispensing with some of these rugs, now that you know they can be hazardous.
- Always use stairways with railings and always hold on to the railing as you climb up or down stairs.

○ Try to avoid using the stairs constantly, by cutting down on unnecessary trips. If you have something to carry upstairs, such as clean laundry, put it by the staircase and take it up with you later, when you have another reason to go upstairs. If there is a suitable room on the main floor of your house, consider moving your bedroom there.

○ Use nonskid rubber mats in the bathtub and shower stall.

○ Make sure floors are completely dry after they're mopped. Don't use a slippery floor wax on your floors.

○ Put away all children's toys and any other extraneous material—even dog bones and toys for your pet—that is just lying around begging to trip someone.

Some physical changes to your house may be needed, such as installing railings on every stairway and grip bars in shower stalls and bathtubs. If there are practical reasons that such changes are not possible (for instance, financial concerns, or if you're renting your home) or until these changes can be made, be extra-careful and vigilant.

Your home first aid kit

If you have never had a home first aid kit handy, setting one up is a wise idea—in addition to being a potential help to you, it comes in handy with kids! If you do have one, this is a good time to review its contents and see whether new items should be added.

Here are the basics of a first aid kit for people with MS:

○ Your favorite ibuprofen brand (for pain relief)

○ Benadryl (for sleep)

○ Bengay or the homeopathic equivalent, Triflora (for muscle pain)

○ Arnica oil (for massaging aches and pains)

○ Hydrogen peroxide

○ Bacitracin

○ Rubbing alcohol

○ Ready-made bandages, such as Band-Aids or another brand, of all sizes

○ Gauze pads or a roll of gauze

○ Waterproof first aid tape
○ Reusable hot and cold packs
○ A&D Ointment or the equivalent
○ A sharps container (for disposal of syringes)

If there is any product you use frequently, keep a duplicate or double on hand. This can save you time and may help you out in a health pinch.

Sharing the bathroom

When a person coping with symptoms of MS shares a bathroom, other members of the household must take care not to make the situation more precarious.

Anyone who shares the bathroom with a person with extra needs should be particularly cautious about cleaning up water spills and about putting towels, soaps, and other bathroom equipment back in their proper place. After taking a bath or shower, everyone in the house should wipe the bathroom floor carefully with a used towel, as an extra precaution against falls.

The bathtub should be washed meticulously after any bath to avoid creating a dangerous slippery surface for a person with MS, especially one who has a hard enough time navigating getting in and out of the tub in the first place. Because new bath oils, bubble baths, and other bath products are often filled with moisturizers, it is extremely important to keep a scrub brush and an antibacterial soap by the tub and to use these to clear the tub of the slippery film that these products leave behind.

Other Safety Tips

○ Wear comfortable low-heel shoes with rubber soles or wear sneakers.
○ Make sure to leave a night-light on to avoid stumbling on any nocturnal visits to the bathroom.
○ Have a grip bar installed in the shower as soon as possible.
○ Cover all exposed heating pipes with protective, heatproof coating to protect from burns.
○ Don't rush anywhere.

The vial of life

It is recommended that elderly people and those with chronic conditions such as MS have a brief list of essential medical information on hand, just in case there is an emergency. Usually, the list is compiled on an index card and contains the person's medications (name and daily dosage), along with contact information for the primary-care physician and any known allergies. Emergency medical personnel call this list the "vial of life." In case of a life-threatening emergency, their having it saves precious time trying to ascertain what medication may be called for or is dangerous to you.

If there's room, the vial of life should also include the name of the hospital your doctor is affiliated with and your insurance carrier and group, or your policy number.

You may want to make up such cards, not only for yourself, but for all members of your household. Keep them in a designated place, and make sure everyone in the house knows where they are and what they're for.

Oddly, perhaps, emergency teams expect to find this information in the butter compartment of the refrigerator door, even though no actual medications are generally included in the vial. If you wish, label the butter compartment "Vial of Life"; put a sign on the refrigerator door indicating that this precious information is inside. Strange as this location may seem, you might as well make another place for the butter. The vial of life is vital for saving time and saving lives.

IN A SENTENCE:

> *Improving home safety is a simple way to avoid injury and to make daily life easier.*

learning

Types and Levels of Disability

EVERYONE WHO is diagnosed with MS wonders what the future will hold, particularly since in certain unenviable cases of progressive MS, severe disabilities may develop. It is these cases we heard about most often before we were diagnosed, and we can't help speculating when we sit in the doctor's office next to someone in a wheelchair. What we do not hear enough about are the many people with MS who never develop any noticeable disability.

While we feel compassion for those with MS who came before us and were unfortunate not to have access to the current disease-modifying therapies, we need also to take heart that we live in a time when more and more treatment options for MS are becoming available. The chances are becoming greater and greater for us all to live a relatively symptom-free and disability-free life for years to come—maybe even for a lifetime.

In some cases, disease-modifying therapies have been known to reverse certain disabilities. For example, Pamela was diagnosed in her thirties, soon after the birth of her second child. With a four-month-old and a three-year-old at home, she found herself blind in one eye, with limited vision in the other, and with severe numbness in her right arm (she is right-handed). Needless to say, she was frightened for herself; in addition, the task of mothering two young children became almost impossible. She had to have help at home to ensure the good care and safety of both her children and herself. After beginning therapy with Avonex, Pamela soon recovered her vision and the use of her arm. After two and a half years, she has had no relapses of vision loss and is happily caring for her children with only her husband's help. There are more and more success stories like this to heed and to inspire you. So focus on these, rather than the dire possibilities that are possible to foresee, but may never occur.

Sometimes the fear of disability may become so intense that a person may let his or her fear begin to affect the course of the life to come. For example, a man diagnosed in his twenties or thirties may feel it would be unfair to a partner to marry, or may make a decision not to start a family because of the possibility of becoming disabled. Letting your fears for the future control your life can be more disabling than any future disability that you may face; it will also add excess and unnecessary stress to your daily life.

For those of you who suspect that reading about possible disabilities may make you more afraid about the future, feel free to skip this section. For those of you who would always rather know than not know, the following is a brief description of possible disabilities that you may face in the future or, unfortunately, are possibly experiencing to some degree now.

Assessing disability

The most common disabilities associated with MS are problems walking and problems with vision.

Walking. An exacerbation or a relapse may lead to difficulty walking; the symptoms involved are gait disorders, balance, and spasticity. These problems generally are minor and resolve themselves with time. During major flare-ups or over the years as MS progresses, some people may need a mechanical aid to assist them in walking: a cane, a walker, or, in severe cases, a wheelchair.

Walking aids can be found at many pharmacies and at surgical-supply stores. You can also look at products online before you go out to buy one, and even order them online if you don't insist on seeing the aid before purchasing it. Another good source is the advertising section "Shopping Mart" in the back of *Inside MS,* the NMSS magazine.

If the thought that you have to use a cane or other walking aid depresses you, keep in mind that even some walking disabilities need not be permanent. Jenny had been diagnosed in her late forties, just as she entered perimenopause. The onset of her MS was sudden and dramatic: she was hospitalized for treatment with cortosteroids, and when she was released, she needed a motorized scooter to get around. Her doctor put her on both a disease-modifying medication and hormone replacement therapy. However, five years after her diagnosis, she was walking well with the assistance of only a cane. She tires easily, but knows to pause and take deep breaths for a few minutes, or to find a chair for a brief rest, before moving on.

Attitude also counts for a great deal when it comes to confronting a walking disability. Bill says, "Anyone walking with a cane who complains about it should stop complaining and be grateful they're walking. That goes for everyone with or without MS." The "bands" Bill often feels constricting his calf muscles and wrapping around his midsection bother him much more than needing the assistance of a cane while walking. Of course, he would rather be walking without assistance, but he is not the type to sit home and sulk.

I have a cane on hand for when I need it. Sometimes, when I'm feeling unsteady, I'll use it to avoid falls and to give a visual warning to let others know to give me the room and time to navigate.

Vision problems. Symptoms such as double vision, image distortion, and periodic partial blindness can worsen and create long-term vision problems, or at worst a permanent partial loss of vision. Legal blindness is not common in MS.

Those who have vision problems often find that these difficulties come and go. While this is annoying, one can at least truly appreciate the preciousness of sight when it is completely available.

Whether a vision problem is temporary or permanent, the first thing to rule out, if it's that serious, is driving.

If you struggle with impaired vision, there are resources available to you. Enhanced large-number dialing phones, magnifying glasses, books with large print, and other such products are available in many places, especially online and in the "Shopping Mart" section of *Inside MS* magazine. You can also order audio books, which you can listen to while walking or relaxing in the evening. All you need is a portable cassette, CD, or MP3 player.

The Descriptive Video Service (DVS) makes it possible to enjoy Public Broadcasting Service programs on TV by providing narrative descriptions of key visual elements in a program at times when the soundtrack pauses. Access this service via the Second Audio Program, now built in to most newer TVs, DVD players, and media systems. You can also rent videos and DVDs from DVS. For contact information, see the Resources section.

Levels of disability

Levels of disability vary and may change when you are dealing with MS. The most frequently used measure of disability is the Kurtzke Disability Status Scale. Introduced in the 1980s and updated since, the Kurtzke Scale may be too strict in terms of what people with MS might face. Nevertheless, the guidelines (abbreviated here) are helpful for those of us facing the possibility of disability due to MS.

1. No disability is defined as no visible disability, with some diminishment of the sense of vibration and some lack of finger-to-nose coordination.
2. Minimal disability involves some weakness or stiffness, minor gait disturbances, and minor problems with vision.
3. Moderate disability involves noticeable sensory loss, increasing *ataxia* (the inability to coordinate muscle movements), bladder issues, and problems with vision.
4. Some severe disability involves increasing stiffness, bladder issues, problems with vision, and other symptoms, but not enough disability to leave a person unable to work or proceed with the normal activities of daily life, though sexual function may be affected.
5. Severe disability is defined as enough disability to make full-time work impossible and involves limitations of mobility, including not being able to walk farther than approximately 500 feet unaided.
6. Such disability is severe enough to involve the use of a cane, crutches, and/or leg braces for walking.
7. This level of disability leaves the person confined to a wheelchair.

Some people with progressive-relapsing MS do become bedridden, but I must repeat that this is not inevitable. It is important to emphasize that even a person with a progressive type of MS who pursues an active course of disease-modifying treatment can live well, with minimal disability, over the course of a lifetime.

IN A SENTENCE:

> *Few have to deal with severe disability in the first year, but those who do will be better prepared to cope if they know what they are facing.*

Starting
a Family

MANY OF the people diagnosed are in their twenties or
thirties, a time of life when we are often involved in starting
families. As it does with countless other aspects of life, MS
becomes a factor for a couple in deciding when to have a first
child, or even subsequent children. While this applies even if
the man is the one with the disease, it is even more important
to consider when the woman is in that position.

The good news is that, even though you may experience
some limitations in your life because of your MS, you need not
let remaining childless be one of them. Study after study has
shown that pregnancy does not affect the future health status
of women with MS. In a study following 178 women, all with
clinically diagnosed MS, there was no difference in the level of
long-term disability, whether the individual had no pregnancies,
a single pregnancy, or two or more. (One may conjecture that
the women who found themselves raising children may have
suffered more frequent bouts of fatigue than the women without children, but obviously child rearing is tiring and sometimes
even arduous, whether or not the parent has MS.)

If you decide to start a family after your diagnosis, you are lucky to have been diagnosed early and in an era in which much more is known about MS and how to treat it than was the case twenty years ago. Back in 1987, during the infamous "Baby M" child-custody case, a neurologist testified that a woman with even a mild form of MS would be playing "Russian roulette" if she were to try to have a child. This doctor's testimony was a detriment to furthering the understanding of MS, and we now know that it was completely inaccurate.

Making the decision

Having children is an affirmation of life and, if you love children, having a family is a pleasure not to be missed. Whether or not to have children is a decision you and your partner must make together, but if one of you has MS, part of the discussion preceding the decision should be with your MS specialist. Women will need to discuss the various medications they will need to stop taking while trying to get pregnant and to discuss how to safely continue their treatment without jeopardizing the fetus during the pregnancy.

If your doctor expresses any reservations about your proceeding to try to have a baby, listen carefully and consider what he or she tells you very carefully. Discuss the issues that the doctor raised with your partner. If you feel these are legitimate concerns, you may want to consider adoption. If not, you have the right and the obligation to seek another opinion, and even to consider changing specialists.

Once again, this is an issue about your life and your identity. You are the one who ultimately has to make the choices regarding your life and who takes responsibility for them. If you and your spouse decide not to try to have a family at someone else's behest, it's possible you may regret your decision for years to come. The emotional stress of that regret could risk jeopardizing your health far more than if you proceed in pursuing your goals in life.

As you consider the facts and advice and weigh your options, remember this: being able to appreciate and take joy in every stage in your children's life is a tremendous motivating factor in staying well. The better your health, the more you will be able to share in their young lives.

If you do have MS and are considering starting a family, you might want to think about keeping the family unit smaller. Raising three or four children is a lot more exhausting than raising one or two, and you do not want to be so fatigued from child rearing that you are constantly at risk for relapses.

Finally, you may be worried about the genetic risk of passing MS on to any children you may have. As has been mentioned earlier, that risk is very low (no more than 1 to 3 percent). If you already have other family members who have MS, or if you have ambivalent feelings about wanting children, that small added risk is something to consider seriously. Otherwise, it probably should not be a deterrent to having a family. After all, life itself is a risk, and all parents-to-be worry about whether they will have a healthy baby.

Getting pregnant

In most cases having MS has nothing to do with your fertility.

If the mother-to-be is the one with MS, issues such as spasticity or discomfort during intercourse may inhibit you and your partner's ability to have sex at the right time—that is, when you are ovulating. If the man is the partner who has MS, issues of the ability to perform may inhibit getting your partner pregnant. In either case, you may simply be able to muddle through. You are just as likely as those without MS to become pregnant in the first six months to a year spent having sexual intercourse without protection. If problems persist or are so serious as to make intercourse painful or impossible, consult a doctor.

If the spastic contractures a woman may experience or if the problems her partner faces inhibit the ability to get pregnant, artificial insemination may be an appropriate option.

Pregnancy and delivery

Generally, your symptoms will not be affected during the actual term of your pregnancy. In fact, you may experience a period of complete and enjoyable remission, dealing only with the common complaints of pregnancy, such as morning sickness and feeling tired. Having MS will also not affect the process of giving birth, nor does it affect having an epidural for pain or in the event of a cesarean section.

After you give birth, your symptoms may be exacerbated. In fact most women who have MS and carry a pregnancy to term do experience one or more relapses once the child is born. Such relapses are probably brought on by the sudden hormonal changes that occur post-pregnancy. This is a period when your doctor will watch you closely and try to combat a relapse with therapies he or she might suggest.

Breastfeeding is safe for mothers with MS.

The first year of life

Consider yourself normal if you and your partner find yourself at an exhausted standoff during much of the first year of your baby's life. Almost all new parents go through this period of adjustment.

Ironically, women and their doctors often worry about exacerbations of MS due to postpartum hormone fluctuations, and these are real concerns, but the biggest drain on the new mom comes from caring for the baby, living with a continually disturbed sleep cycle, and adjusting to all the additional chores that come with a newborn.

To try to keep yourself healthy while you are keeping your growing baby healthy (and to assist in keeping your relationship with your partner healthy and functioning), you will need to get your rest. And in order to do that, you will need some help. All new mothers need help, but a woman with MS who has a new baby needs it even more.

Depending on the family budget, this help might come in the form of full-time or part-time baby care, or friends and family. If members of your family live nearby, discuss arrangements for baby-sitting during your pregnancy. (By the way, this is a great way to allow your parents or your in-laws to get involved with their grandchild and to assist you in your daily fight with MS.)

When you are first home from the hospital with your newborn, everyone will want to come visit. Don't let this be a burden to you. If family members agreed beforehand to baby-sit, go to your bedroom and lie down for a brief rest while they're there cooing at your child—try not to make tea and have a social call, and no matter what, don't use this precious downtime to clean the kitchen.

As your baby grows, and you adjust to having a new member of the family, you'll also adjust to the give-and-take between you and the unpaid baby-sitters, be they family members or friends. Eventually, you'll want to use some of your time off, so to speak, to get out of the house and get back to having a life of your own. This could take the form of getting back to work, exercising, or lunching out with another friend.

If you had been working full-time before your delivery, do everything you can to take as much maternity leave as possible. Use this time not only to get to know your new baby, but also to reestablish your health regimen and get the rest you need. If your employer will allow you a short leave without pay in addition to your maternity benefits, and your family budget allows it, take the added time. It will do both you and your baby good. As you prepare to go back to work, find out whether it's possible for you to get a "flex time" work schedule; try to do so, since you will enjoy the extra time at home with the baby and it may reduce your child-care costs.

Many couples report that it helps to devise an at-home schedule as well. A working partner should relieve the stay-at-home parent for a few hours each evening, and for a longer period on the weekend. You both need some time by yourself to relax.

When I spoke to Gemma and Nancy, they had a one-year-old named Ruby. Three years before, Nancy had been diagnosed with MS. Both these women were in their thirties and as life partners they wanted to start a family. After a series of conversations, they decided that Gemma would be the biological parent to avoid any medical risk a pregnancy might pose for Nancy. The pregnancy was successful, Ruby is healthy, and so are Nancy and Gemma.

Nancy has still not stopped thinking about having her own biological child. She has been doing well with her symptoms, although sometimes she does have to walk with a cane. She explained that she loved Ruby so much, why not love two children? They're still in the thinking stages, but the whole family is happy with their good fortune, including Ruby, who sleeps through the night.

Interestingly, the issues the two women have about parenting are the same as those of heterosexuals when one partner has MS. Gemma thinks Nancy should do more baby care. Nancy feels she does as much as she can, given that she also must cope with her symptoms, including fatigue and issues of spasticity. This is a family in progress, managing well with a new baby and a parent with MS. Whatever your own partnership is or will be, you can manage too.

IN A SENTENCE:

> *If you want to have children, your MS usually will not affect your chances for a healthy pregnancy and a healthy baby.*

learning

Improving Your Memory and Powers of Concentration

COGNITION REFERS to such mental skills as memory, planning, and the ability to exercise judgment and foresight. In the past, complaints from those with MS regarding concentration issues or memory loss were often disregarded, dismissed, or attributed to dullness or emotional issues. However, it's now known that MS may affect cognition in one third of those diagnosed; about 10 percent of those diagnosed may in fact face serious problems related to cognition.

Memory

Whenever I am forgetful, I adamantly insist to myself that it has to do with encroaching middle age, and not my MS. Nevertheless, I recognize there may be some creative denial at work here, and I don't let it stop me from practicing exercises to improve my mental agility and keep my memory functioning as well as possible.

If you have been diagnosed at a reasonably young age, in your twenties or thirties, the idea of memory loss may seem quite foreign. Keep your memory in great shape by practicing memorization exercises—for instance, commit the phone numbers of friends to memory, rather than relying on the speed-dial button, or, with cellular phones, the stored numbers.

One of the best ways to cope with any memory problems is to make small compensations in your day-to-day routine. These adjustments will keep you organized and keep you from forgetting anything of importance. Despite how I just advised younger people with MS against relying on speed dial, it's a great device for people in their forties and fifties—relying on it to recall your frequently dialed numbers frees space in your memory bank for other things.

Another great gadget is the PalmPilot. Having everything—schedule, reminders, phone numbers, addresses—stored in one place is a good and necessary crutch. Back up all the data on your PalmPilot on your home computer, since otherwise, if you forget it someplace or if your purse, backpack, or briefcase is stolen, you will be at a loss.

A simple wall calendar in the home, posted in the kitchen or near a phone, is a good low-tech backup for important dates and events. As for important phone numbers, take the time to exercise your writing hand and write them down in your personal phone book, Filofax, or on a piece of paper you post on a bulletin board in the kitchen or home office.

Another good way to outsmart a faulty memory is to write notes to yourself and keep lists. For example, if tomorrow is a busy day with a number of appointments and errands, make a list for yourself the night before; this will ensure a worry-free night's sleep and prevent your forgetting a meeting or chore in the morning. Also, use a notepad at a convenient location (for instance, the kitchen or front hall) to keep a running shopping list. Write down the item you need as soon as your supply is low.

You may also want to write reminders on Post-its and stick them on the refrigerator, like Rebecca, who has two school-age children and works part-time. "I spend a lot of time in the kitchen," she says. "So I've made my own lemonade out of a lemon, I guess. Notes about doctors' appointments, birthday parties, packing the kids' lunches for a field trip, dinner dates, which days are shot days . . . they're all up on the fridge. When they lose their stickiness, I just write a new one. I use multicolored ones because it's prettier." Self-stick notes also work well on a wall calendar or the bathroom mirror.

To remind yourself to take a particular medication in the morning, leave the pill bottle on the bathroom counter in plain sight with a glass next to it for water.

Another memory trick is to remind yourself out loud of your plans for the day. Since others might wonder why you're talking to yourself, this technique is best reserved for the times when you're alone. It has worked for my friend Bill, who says, "I have found that if I vocalize my thoughts, they tend to 'stick' better than if I just plan something out in my head."

When you are at work or out, keep a notebook with you at all times and write down everything you need to remember. If it's not convenient to write something down, take off your watch and put it on your other wrist or change a ring to another finger. Later, when you do a double take and ask yourself why you did that, you'll jog your memory and remember the item and, this time, write it down. Another way to remind yourself of something important is to call home and leave yourself a message on the answering machine. If you are a true techie, you may want to purchase a mini-tape recorder and dictate important information to yourself during the day. Everyone will simply think you're a doctor or an undercover agent!

Concentration

If you have trouble getting focused on a new task or staying focused on the matter at hand, whether in the office, out running errands, or at home, you may be having a concentration problem caused at least in part by your MS. Problems involving concentration may even affect your ability to communicate, which can be terribly frustrating, particularly if you are a highly social person. The noise and bustle of a crowd, even at a party you were looking forward to, can overwhelm you.

If you have concerns regarding your capacity to concentrate and related issues, discuss them with your doctor. If your issues are serious, he or she may recommend a speech and language therapist, a psychologist, or a neuropsychologist. There are also some exercises you might want to do to help yourself function more effectively in maintaining your concentration and in communicating.

Jonathan is a computer programmer who worried after his diagnosis whether he would be able to stay in his chosen field. He tried an exercise, suggested in a self-help book, of counting backward out loud from ten to zero. "I started doing it automatically. I guess it's like counting sheep, only backward and for the opposite reason. I'm nearly a year into my MS, but I do think it helps. It's a kind of meditation, but, if nothing else, it keeps me from thinking bad thoughts."

When people have concentration problems, the interruptions of daily life are even more annoying. Another way to improve your powers of concentration is to set aside time during the day to read an article, poem, or report from beginning to end. This means dispensing with television, loud music, cell phones, etc. Treated in this way, reading becomes a form of meditation. If your schedule allows, lengthen your uninterrupted reading time to at least half an hour. Such constructive solitude will help you concentrate more thoroughly and for longer periods of time. It will also allow you to experience a peaceful time.

Speaking of meditation, both meditation and yoga are excellent ways to help improve your concentration, as well as lower your anxiety level. Anxiety can often get in the way of concentration.

Maintaining your concentration while out in public or among larger groups can be difficult. At parties, if you're in a loud and crowded room and can't hear or concentrate, excuse yourself and find a rest room. Once you gather your forces and return to the party, look for a quieter corner of the room, or take a friend outside for a brief walk and a one-on-one conversation.

Regarding social obligations, you should talk through your issues involving large gatherings or crowds with your spouse, partner, or date, or the friend you go with, and come to an agreement about strategies. With clear communication ahead of time, neither of you will feel guilt, blame the other for "ruining" the evening, or feel offended. Adapt creatively to the social situation at hand. Make sure the person knows that you may start feeling very overwhelmed and have to leave the function early. With a family member, discuss how you'll get home separately.

IN A SENTENCE:

> *To maintain cognitive abilities, work on your memory skills and your powers of concentration.*

MONTH 9

living

Updating Your
Medical Situation

YOU'VE MADE it through nine months of living with MS. Whether you have relapsing-remitting MS, primary-progressive MS, or another type, take a moment to pat yourself on the back for how well you've done so far.

This is a good time to evaluate your entire medical situation. About this time, you will probably be asked to come in for another examination by your MS specialist. If you were ignoring other medical matters during the first months after your diagnosis, you should have adjusted to your new routine enough to make those appointments now. And I'll also give you some more tips on avoiding infections, which, as you know, can rev up your immune system and thus exacerbate your MS symptoms.

Your MS checkup

Besides discussing any new symptoms and your progress with your MS specialist, you may find it helpful to use your next checkup to take measure of your treatment plan and your medical team.

If you are still unable to deal with the side effects of the medication you are taking, you should discuss changing your medication. Which medication you're switching from or to is important, so review the merits of each with your doctor. Also keep in mind that the goal remains the same: treating your MS as well as possible while keeping your overall health as good as possible.

If you are having any trouble coping with your symptoms, this should be part of your discussion with your doctor. You need to be frank and direct. Remember that your doctor is there to help you—don't be shy about describing your symptoms, and don't worry that you are taking up too much of your doctor's time.

If you are not happy with your doctor, consider whether you should find another specialist. You can ask other members of your medical team for a referral, or seek recommendations from others with MS.

On the other hand, if you are satisfied, it's always nice to thank your doctor for taking such good care of you.

On My Broken Arm

YES, WE have enough to deal with, but even when you are coping with MS, life could care less. This summer I took my son to Idaho, where my recently deceased father was born and raised and where I had skated at Sun Valley as a competitive figure skater. While I was skating, I had to avoid hitting a little girl on the ice and I fell, breaking my arm.

I spent much of the summer in a cast to the elbow, but after the first two weeks of pain, I made friends with my cast rather than fighting it. I was still able to give myself my shot, and I got kudos for being in great shape and keeping my bones strong. It wasn't easy, but sometimes it's great to know you are doing well in a lot of ways, not just in dealing with your major issue—MS.

Don't ignore other medical conditions

You have learned that having MS isn't the one thing that defines you. This condition doesn't limit what you can do with your life; the flip side of the coin is that just because you have MS doesn't mean that you are free from paying attention to other medical conditions. Your overall health is important and you are still susceptible to the same kinds of medical ailments that other people your age commonly get.

By now, you've settled into a routine and are no longer feeling so overwhelmed by your new status. If you've been putting off other medical appointments, now is the time to pay attention to all issues that may affect your health.

Begin by having a regular, overall medical checkup with your primary-care physician or internist. This is particularly important if you have any other conditions, such as high blood pressure or high cholesterol.

Make sure to ask for a regular blood analysis, to ensure that any new medications you're taking to combat MS aren't causing side effects elsewhere. If you are a woman, see your gynecologist for regular checkups and Pap smears.

Make a dental appointment and stick to a schedule of routine cleanings and checkups. There is no need to fear the X-rays dentists use to check for cavities—they have only a low level of radiation.

Speaking of your mouth, if you have gum disease or had it in the past, see your periodontist.

If you are a woman approaching forty or over forty, regular mammograms are useful to screen for breast cancer.

Preventing viral infections

Your MS specialist will probably be constantly recommending regular checkups with your internist and may seem overly concerned with any complaints of fever or illness you might broach. The reason for this concerted medical effort is to help you avoid viral infection.

A viral infection is one of the only factors that has been proven to worsen symptoms or increase the risk of a relapse in relapsing-remitting MS. As many as one fourth to one half of MS relapses are triggered by an initial viral infection, which then calls the immune system to action. As you know, when you have MS, your immune system is wired to work *against* you as well as *for* you.

The best way to avoid the risk of relapse is to take precautions to avoid viral infections whenever possible. Such precautions include:

O Getting enough sleep and rest. If you are run-down, you are at greater risk of contracting a viral infection.

○ Avoiding contact with friends who have infections. For instance, if you have a dinner date with someone with flulike symptoms, politely reschedule.

○ Getting a flu shot during flu season. There are no studies that show that getting the flu vaccine increases the risk of relapse.

○ If you have a persistent cough and your physician feels you are at risk for bronchitis, taking the recommended antibiotic and completing the course of treatment. It's better than courting pneumonia and will help minimize your risk of relapse.

Preventing bladder infections

Bladder infections are a common, annoying ailment. They occur most commonly when the urine is not acidic enough and when voiding is incomplete. While a bladder infection can be easily cured with antibiotics, it's preferable not to get one in the first place. Here are some things you can do to avoid this sort of infection:

○ Make sure you go to the bathroom often enough, in order to avoid storing urine in the bladder for long periods of time.

○ To make sure you've voided completely, wait an extra moment or two standing in front of or sitting on the toilet, to see if another dribble of urine comes out. There's no need to hurry away from the toilet— we rush enough in this world, and this rushing "instinct" often has negative consequence on many aspects of our health care, including our bathroom habits. My motto is "Don't rush to flush."

○ If, in a routine abdominal sonogram, your doctor finds you are retaining urine, he or she might consider catheterization, either in the doctor's office or at home. While catheterization may be uncomfortable, it is a painless procedure that is easy to perform and is worth the effort in order to painful prevent bladder infections.

○ Women should void before and after intercourse to eliminate the buildup of bacteria.

○ To increase the acid content of your urine and ward off infections, drink plenty of cranberry juice. Use unsweetened cranberry juice. If it is too tart, try adding some Stevia (the herbal substitute for sweeteners) or mix the juice with water. If you hate cranberry juice, you can obtain cranberry tablets or caplets at your local health-food store or pharmacy.

○ If you feel any irritation while urinating, call your physician right away. The sooner an infection is treated, the less likely it will activate your immune system to such a degree that you then experience a worsening of symptoms or a relapse.

If you are diagnosed with a bladder infection, your doctor will prescribe an antibiotic. Make sure you take the antibiotic as directed and that you finish the full prescription, to guarantee that all the offending bacteria have been eliminated and that you will not experience a recurrent infection.

All those doctors' visits

One dubious distinction you are no doubt acquiring in managing MS is an intimate knowledge of medical-office waiting rooms. Sitting there waiting can be tedious, so here are some tips to make the waiting game less of a drag:

○ Make your appointments early in the day. This way it's hard for the doctor to be behind in seeing patients.

○ If you feel anxious about a certain problem or condition, ask the office assistant to contact you if there is a cancellation, in case you can make an earlier appointment.

○ Call your doctor's office before you leave for your appointment to see how far behind, if at all, he or she is running. If your appointment is for noon and the doctor is running fifteen minutes late, for instance, ask the assistant whether you can come in at 12:15 *without* losing your slot (that is, without falling behind the person with the 12:30 appointment, who might arrive before you).

○ If you are concerned about remembering everything that happens during your examination, bring a friend or family member with you.

○ Always bring something to read while you're waiting. The magazines in doctors' offices are rarely current. My advice is to bring with you all the magazines or catalogs that you haven't gotten around to reading. If you finish them, leave them behind for other patients.

IN A SENTENCE:

> *Your health consists of much more than MS—don't neglect your overall well-being.*

learning

Other Medication Options

BY NOW it is safe to say you will have adjusted to your medication, *if you are going to adjust*. If you are still having trouble with unpleasant side effects and are unable to say enthusiastically that you have felt better or seen signs of improvement in your physical functions, it's time to have a serious talk with your doctor. Make notes before you go to your appointment. If you want to keep trying but have problems with the frequency of self-injections, let your MS specialist know you're determined to go forward with treatment.

Switching medications

There are many options in the medical treatment of MS, and your doctor is as committed to finding the right one for you as you are. Regardless of which of the four major disease-modifying medications you're on—Copaxone, Avonex, Rebif, or Betaseron—any one of these is usually a viable option. You can switch to another one, which may have fewer side effects that are really bothersome to you, or a more pleasing means or frequency of injection.

Novantrone

Another drug to consider switching to, if your condition warrants, is Novantrone, a powerful immune system suppressant. This medication works well to slow down the relentless course of any of the progressive types of MS; in particular, it reduces neurologic disability. It also helps people dealing with any relapsing-remitting MS of a type that seems to be advancing too quickly.

Novantrone is administered intravenously once every three months. Obviously, the advantage of having only four doses a year is somewhat offset by the disadvantage of the way it's given.

The drug is not intended for anyone who is managing well in treatment and experiencing a limited number of symptoms and relapses. That's because there is a lifetime dose limit. You can take the drug only so many times and then you must stop. The reason for this is that the medication can cause arrhythmia (irregular heartbeat) and damage the heart over time.

Other side effects include nausea, alopecia (hair loss), menstrual disorders (including amenorrhea), urinary-tract infections, diarrhea or constipation, and stomatitis (inflammation of the oral cavity).

If you have progressive MS, or if you are feeling discouraged by a noticeable physical decline from RRMS, discuss the pros and cons of going on Novantrone for a while with your MS specialist.

Other medications to treat MS

By now, it's clear that Bill, who rides his bike everywhere when he's at home but also travels as far afield as India, is a very colorful character. When I last caught up with him, he told me he had consented to undergo a somewhat radical treatment program for MS that includes low doses of chemotherapy. He's had one dose and soon planned to go for another MRI to see if the chemo has helped retard the demyelination from his progressive MS. Bill said, "I'm somewhat skeptical. I need to see the MRI to convince myself it's worth it to go through this again. I have a theory that anything with any power must also have a deleterious effect. You just have to decide

Depression

REGARDLESS OF whether you're sticking with your original disease-modifying medication or switching, you may at times feel depressed by your continuing fight with MS. This is perfectly natural—feeling down is nothing to be ashamed of. People can become depressed for any reason, including very small reasons. You have a valid reason to be depressed.

Sometimes, however, depression gets bad enough that it inhibits your ability to function and keep fighting the disease. Be on the alert for signs of moderate or serious depression (share them with your loved ones, who may notice a change in you before you yourself do). Symptoms of depression include lack of motivation, additional fatigue, listlessness, the inability to keep up a daily schedule, a further loss of energy, loss of appetite, and more problems with sleeping than usual.

If you do feel depressed, don't let it conquer your will to manage your illness. Get over being embarrassed about feeling bad. Remember that any level of depression will increase your fatigue level, so there is a practical reason to get help. You do not have to go it alone. Get help if you need it. Talking to a minister, rabbi, or therapist might help; in more serious cases, a psychiatrist or other physician might give you a short prescription for an antidepressant medication.

if the benefits are worth the cost." Regardless of the outcome, Bill is happy —in fact, he says he's happier than he was before he finally got his diagnosis. Part of the reason is in fact that he is exploring an experimental technique. "It's a good thing, you see," he explained. "I have become curious again."

While I haven't been able to find out anything about the treatment procedure Bill is following, I mention this to inspire you to keep open to new possibilities that might work for your individual case.

IN A SENTENCE:

> *If your disease-modifying medication is not satisfactory, switch to a different one.*

Your Relationships: What's Changed, What's Stayed the Same

BY NOW, you've had time to examine how living with your MS affects your interactions with your spouse, family, and friends. In fact, during their first year living with MS, many people report that some of the relationships in their lives change.

It's not only okay but also probably inevitable that some of the relationships you've had in the past are changing now. In some cases, the change can even be liberating. You may even find that having MS has helped you be stronger about making decisions about how you deal with the important people in your life.

It's not a matter of picking fights with old friends and family members, but you may have noticed that some of those you hold dear have stood staunchly by you while others have become also-rans. If the latter has happened, and you have done all that you can to resolve a difficult situation that remains untenable, accept that this is how things have turned out. As you contemplate the change in the relationship, let go of any guilt or anxiety, be patient with yourself, and remind yourself that right now your priority is to nurture your own good health.

Family

My research for this book led me to many earlier treatments of the subject, including some published a few years back. I was surprised to find that several of these books advocated that the family take a "tough love" approach to dealing with the patient. They suggested not catering to the person with MS all day. They advised against focusing the entire family's attention on the one "suffering" from MS.

This strikes me as wrongheaded denial of the facts: remember that more women than men get the disease, so it stands to reason that the person in the family with MS is often a young wife and mother who is actively running a household, helping her husband and children organize their lives, and in many cases holding down a full-time job as well. Isn't it more likely that it goes the other way around, and that instead of not being catered to, she needs extra support and understanding? The woman with MS needs her family's help as she juggles housekeeping, being a loving wife and mother, and managing her disease.

If you're a woman with MS, make sure your immediate family doesn't ignore your condition. Children should be entrusted with household chores appropriate to their age. Your husband also needs to chip in with the housework—maybe he's not a good cook, but he can do the shopping or the laundry, or give the kids their baths.

When I feel overextended or taken for granted, it bothers me how much my family relies on me in physical ways. I realize it's possible I don't ask for help often enough. The truth is I appear functional, and since people often judge a book by its cover, my family continues to rely on me a bit too much.

This may be a case of do as I say, not as I do, but talk to your family regularly about things they can do to pitch in to help. The bottom line is that while we do not want to be treated as if we were Fabergé eggs, nor do we want those around us to expect us to be superwomen. Or supermen—men with MS feel similar pressures, especially if they are the sole breadwinner in the family.

Your spouse or partner

The first year of living with MS is never easy. It goes without saying that it's a tremendous burden on you, but if you're in a long-term, committed relationship it's also something for your husband, wife, or partner to adjust to. Regardless of good intentions, sometimes your spouse or partner has exceptional difficulties adjusting to your diagnosis.

I know this to be true, because it happened to me. A little over a year before I was diagnosed with MS, I had just gotten remarried. We were having the usual difficulties adjusting to living together—there's a lot of truth in the cliché that "the first year of marriage is hell"—but after I took the fall down stairs that was mentioned earlier, I resolved to keep the peace at home. I concentrated on trying to figure out what was wrong with me and receive a definitive diagnosis of something, anything. For that spring and most of the summer, my mission was my health.

Soon after my MS specialist confirmed the diagnosis and explained my disease to me, he asked about my personal life. I explained to him that my husband had not seemed to believe me when I told him I had MS. I do not blame my husband for this. Just as it may be hard for us to believe that we have this often invisible disease, it can be equally hard, if not harder, for those who care for us to understand and accept the diagnosis. In any event, Dr. Sadiq suggested he meet with both of us.

These meetings with my specialist did the trick. My husband accepted the diagnosis from this doctor, who was an expert in the field. Dr. Sadiq was brimming with optimism about researching new treatment options and finding a cure. His attitude gave both my husband and me hope. And his ability to communicate clearly and calmly about what must often be a depressing disease seemed to help my husband and me begin really communicating about my condition.

I have been fortunate enough to be relatively asymptomatic, but after those conferences with my doctor, my husband was far more willing to try to understand what he might not have been able to see in regard to my condition. When I found myself thinking, "Well, he just doesn't get it," I reminded myself that if I didn't ask for what I needed, and if I didn't say how I was feeling or describe a certain symptom that was plaguing me, I could not expect sympathy or understanding from him.

Establishing a give-and-take of communication with a spouse or partner who has problems grappling with your diagnosis is vital. More often than not, it is you—the person with MS—who has to take the initiative to start the process, but the end result—mutual understanding and renewed trust and love—is well worth it.

If you have an imperfect relationship, as most of us do, but feel that it is still fundamentally sound, work at improving it. This kind of work is not necessarily stressful (it's only nonproductive work that adds stress).

If you find you are having difficulties and your MS specialist is not available to explain your condition to your partner, seek the help of a couple's therapist. A therapist can help assess the issues bothering you and your partner and help you along the way to better communication and understanding. The sooner you manage the repair work on your relationship, the more supported you will feel in your effort to cope with MS physically and emotionally.

Getting out of a marriage or long-term relationship

A diagnosis of MS will test any relationship, and studies do show that the rate of divorce is higher among those with MS. As we make our vows and state "for better or for worse," we are sincere about sticking to the deal we are making. A young couple starting out may be prepared for the usual issues and problems of living together and making ends meet, but few are prepared for a health crisis of this magnitude. Some couples are up to the test and some are not.

If you have been in your marriage or committed relationship for some time and have already experienced too many compromises and too much disappointment, a diagnosis of MS may be the catalyst that prompts you and your partner to part ways. Divorce is a terribly stressful process, but if your marriage or long-term partnership is satisfying neither of you, the stress of the relationship may be worse for you than the stress of divorce. If you are the person with MS, not the partner, you should make sure you discuss the situation with your MS specialist before taking any major steps to change your personal life.

People in the midst of divorce, with or without a debilitating disease, often tend to be at odds constantly. Beware of this, since you will need to avoid as much stress as possible to stay well. That separation and divorce arrangements should proceed as peacefully as possible is obvious, even though in the real world this advice may not help.

My own marriage had become very difficult and enervating. I spoke to my specialist about this often. He could see the toll the marriage was taking on my overall health and that I was unhappy. My doctor very much wanted to alleviate the stress that coping with the relationship was causing. He even met with the two of us yet another time to try to reach my husband regarding the necessity of helping me or at least allowing me to take special care of my health.

Unfortunately, my husband still wasn't able to truly understand that I had a serious condition I had to cope with every day.

Once I realized that the situation was not healthy for me, I took the necessary steps to end it.

Taking the "Ugh" Out of Dating after Divorce

Once I was divorced, I was so busy feeling lucky that I wasn't even thinking about dating. Then came the world of romance. Needless to say, I'd forgotten a lot, but as with riding that bicycle, you remember very quickly. You also soon recall that it's not that much fun or that easy to get right. I had a few bumpy rides where I made the obvious mistakes—trusting too much, following his lead too easily, letting him make the moves and the rules, and, perhaps most painful of all, feeling grateful for the attention (as if that alone were enough!). I soon learned to stick up for my dating rights and formulated the following rules to protect myself from getting hurt emotionally and, just as important, from getting exhausted!

The New Rules (for MS and dating)

1. Stay away from late nights. For obvious reasons, you want to avoid exhaustion. It's bad for your health. Instead of dates that last much too late, consider these strategies: meet for lunch and an afternoon movie or walk in the park; meet after work for an early drinks date; and if you like each other and decide to pursue a sexual relationship, suggest making love in the early morning—many people find this a sexy indulgence, and this gives you the freedom to conk out in the evening if your body tells you you must.
2. Tell when the telling is right.

3. Speak up before there's a problem.
4. If you inject yourself, don't make a date for the same day, or at least build in lots of time for yourself around giving yourself the shot.
5. If you break up, remember: no guilt, and it's not you. You're only guilty of anything if you're not taking care of yourself.
6. Take your time getting involved.
7. Most important, put your health first.

What makes a relationship work?

In general, the couple that stays together with and through MS already has good lines of communication open. The person diagnosed will disclose the illness right away, and the couple will face the possibilities during the first year, and beyond, as a strong unit.

Here are some guidelines of good communication that have benefited couples who have done well with MS (also note that, when these guidelines are broadened beyond the specifics of MS, each one can be applied to strengthen any long-term relationship).

The person who has been diagnosed makes the decision not to burden the partner with the medical issues pertaining to MS. He or she handles these medical issues primarily with the MS expert, although information is shared with the partner. The principle here is that the responsibility for treating the disease does not lie with the partner. Rather, information is shared to maintain intimacy. "This is what is going on with me," you say to your partner, and he or she listens, is sympathetic, and understands what you're confronting.

As much as possible the extended family, close friends, and the community are included in a support network. These couples realize that you cannot do it alone.

They learn not to make MS part of the relationship. For them it is a medical issue to be dealt with, not something that defines how they treat each other or relate to each other. The less MS takes center stage, the better.

The couples strive to make sure a deep and nurturing sexual relationship remains part of the partnership, even when this might begin to take a little ingenuity. The couples that survive together seem to realize that asking for help and allowing pleasure to continue to be a part of life is the best way to live together, whatever the medical issues may be.

Your children

Things may or may not change much in terms of how your kids are coping with your new issue; it depends on how well you're doing, their ages, and so many other intangible factors. Savvy children may react by watching you a lot or ignoring you a lot . . . you never know.

If you haven't already done so, now is a good time to revisit the subject of MS and ask how they think it's all going. If you are doing well, that's a good way to introduce the topic. If you've had relapses or lots of symptoms, you might begin by sharing any encouraging words you've had from your doctor on how things are going.

If you do have symptoms that have changed the way the household runs and works, the conversation should involve asking for your family's patience, as well as their help, and telling them that you are still committed to fighting the good fight.

Patrick, my friend Peggy's son, is one of the children who handle the situation amazingly well. Peggy and I had made a lunch date when her son unexpectedly came home from college for the weekend. She asked if she could bring him along because they didn't have a lot of time to visit. Of course, I said, but asked, "What if we start going on about MS?" She said, "Patrick doesn't care. He knows more about it than I do." She was right. The first thing he said to me was, "I hope you're on one of the disease-modifying treatments." Talk about a good adjustment! In fact, when he's home, and Peggy isn't feeling all that well or brave, he gives his mother her shot.

When I spoke to Fred, he had just attended his daughter's Bas Mitzvah. He had been managing progressive MS for about ten years, but had reached a stage where he had to walk with a cane and sometimes found himself unable to get up out of a chair without assistance.

While the party was being planned, Fred became worried about dancing at the Bas Mitzvah. One day, since he felt this apprehension was too stressful, he asked his daughter, "How would you feel if I said I wasn't up to dancing with you at your party?"

"Dad, it's fine," she answered. "You'll be there. That's all that matters to me." These are words any father would want to hear. They hugged a lot on the day of the big event, and his daughter danced with her uncles. So far, Fred is still doing well, and his daughter's support only helps!

In my own case, my son and I had the unfortunate duty of attending the funeral of the mother of one of his best friends in school. On the walk home, my son took my hand, even though holding Mom's hand was a thing of the past. He said, "Mom, don't get cancer. . . . Well, I guess I can't say that, but don't die from cancer." After a few moments, he added, referring to my MS, "Oh yeah, you have enough to deal with. And don't die from that either." I promised him I wouldn't.

Around that time, I noticed that while I always gave myself my shot when he was out of the room, he seemed to want to hang around. Eventually, he asked me if he could tap the bubbles out of the syringe with the pen I always use to do that. He has a great interest in science and medicine, so I wasn't all that surprised. These days he keeps me company when he's home on shot day, although he skips watching the actual injection. I'm grateful, and I'm proud of him.

Nonetheless, none of us can expect our kids to be perfect. Your own children will continue to hurt your feelings, because most of the time they don't even know they're doing it. Just because you have a life-threatening (though not fatal) condition doesn't mean you're exempt from being taken for granted, teased, ignored, and not listened to by your children. It happens to all of us parents, whether we have MS or not.

Hot-tempered, needy, or desperate friends

The best friends are precious resources and it's affirming when they're there to support you as you fight MS. However, there are other kinds of friends too, people with their own issues who can be "high maintenance." In this first year of adjusting to your diagnosis, you may discover that some of the latter kind of friends fall by the wayside.

If someone has always asked you for favors, leaned on you, or expected you to come through—without similar benefits flowing your way—this may be the time to cut your losses. Chances are this is not a person you can rely on when times are rough. If you feel less inclined to call such a person, that's okay; in fact, you may have already noticed that the person calls you less often since you told him or her your news.

Admittedly, it can be difficult to end a friendship, or even to tone it down, but you are acting in your own best interest. Being a doormat for your needy friends is not a position your health allows you to be in anymore. If someone appears to be about to step on you, walk away.

This is what I decided to do when I didn't respond to a strange letter that arrived from a self-involved old boyfriend of mine who lives on the West Coast. Among those loved ones I told soon after my diagnosis was another friend who lives in California but often travels to New York City. It seemed like the right thing to do, since I was discovering that leaving so much of what's going on in my life out of the conversation is very stressful. However, I did specifically ask him *not* to tell our mutual friend, this erratic ex-beau.

Imagine my surprise when a few months later, I received a strange, garbled letter from said beau, with a picture of his new son. It was all about the difficulty of the terrible "battle" I was facing and the "burden" I was bearing, and, of course, the requisite self-congratulatory words about his beautiful boy and his immense well-being. I tore envelope, note, and photo in almost exact halves and threw the whole confusing mess away.

The lesson here is that you can never know what those you tell will do with the information. Some trade information as a form of currency. Others will honor your confidences. Telling others will be an imperfect process with at least some unexpected reactions and other surprises occurring over time. There is no way around this, so shrug your shoulders and go forward.

IN A SENTENCE:

> *Modify or, if possible, eliminate the relationships that are not helping you cope with your MS.*

learning

Finding
Support Groups

SUPPORT GROUPS can be a great source of comfort. Regardless of the many different ways in which the disease presents itself and in which it progresses, no one understands what you are going through as you fight MS more than someone else with MS. Talking with people who can immediately key into your description of a symptom or relate to how you felt during a relapse gives a special kind of support.

A support group can take many forms. It can be as simple and small as you and a friend who also has MS. It can have regularly scheduled meetings, weekly or monthly, or it can be an online community, with message boards and chats, that some people visit daily and others go to only when the mood strikes them. Whatever type of support group you find, talking to people who have what you have and know what you know can be a very affirming experience.

Personally, I am the keep-it-to-yourself, get-on-with-business type, and I didn't know what I was missing until I began to interview other people with MS for this book. Talking to these folks was like swimming in a cool brook after having been walking in a parched desert. And, trust me, the camaraderie went both ways. I've kept in touch with a lot of them, and sharing my experiences and ideas—and hearing theirs—has proven to be an enormous help.

The fact that for some of us the symptoms are invisible and for others they are all too obvious can make people on either side of the line uncomfortable in an MS support group. If you are walking around just fine, you may feel guilty in front of those who aren't. And if you are already using a cane, or a scooter, or a wheelchair, you may not want to look back. Partly for this reason, MS support groups online have become enormously popular. In addition, as you find yourself feeling more and more comfortable with the voices you talk to on the Internet, you will feel the freedom to say what you need to say and tell the truth completely. Sometimes, there is nothing like anonymity to allow you to be honest.

In-person support groups

You can stumble across a support group very easily once you make your diagnosis known. Maybe you already have a friend who has MS, or more likely someone you know has a friend with the disease and introduces the two of you. You'll also meet others with MS at your specialist's office, and it's possible some of you will decide to meet for coffee or lunch and share ideas about coping with the disease.

Many local chapters of the national MS organizations also have support groups. For example, call the National Multiple Sclerosis Society at 800-344-4867 (800-FIGHTMS).

And you can also find them through churches, clubs, community centers, and other locally based organizations. In my neighborhood in Manhattan, for instance, there is even a support group at the Lesbian and Gay Community Services Center, which serves all of New York City, for homosexuals with MS.

Support groups are easy to find by asking around or making a few phone calls. Your doctor may also have tips on locating a local group. Of course, you can also use the Internet to search for in-person groups, as described below.

On the Internet

The Internet provides easy access to locating support groups, those meeting face-to-face in your local area as well as online communities, message boards, chat rooms, and discussion groups. Here's a rundown on sites you can visit to find a support group that's convenient and right for you.

The National Multiple Sclerosis Society is very active in organizing support groups on the local level. A visit to its website (www.nationalmssociety. org) can lead the user to local support groups. Simply click on "My Community" and you will be taken to a page asking you what state you live in. Clicking on the state will lead you to contact information concerning support groups in your state. The information provided is very helpful, including such details as contact names, phone numbers, meeting locations and times, and special MS events for those wishing to become more involved with supporting the MS community.

The NMSS also hosts a very active online community of support. Chat rooms provide continuous online support groups one can access at any hour, and message boards allow one to both give and seek out information and support.

MSWorld (www.msworld.org) connects individuals with multiple sclerosis online as well. There are a number of chat rooms to choose from, as well as message boards and e-mail groups. This site is efficiently designed and organized and thus easy to use. First clicking on "Chat" and then clicking on "Chat Schedule" will provide a list of different chat rooms, providing details about the main topics and focus of each room with another click of your mouse. In addition, each state has its own chat room, allowing for more regionalized discussion. Make sure to check meeting times for online discussions in the various chat rooms.

Another good site belongs to the Multiple Sclerosis Foundation (www.msfacts.org). Clicking on "Support Groups" will lead you to a map where a click on your state will summon up detailed information about support groups and upcoming MS events in your area.

The International MS Support Foundation has support groups in many states and Canadian provinces. Its website (www.ms-supportgroup.org) gives you the opportunity to volunteer to start a support group in your area.

Last but not least, there is the Betaseron: Patients and Caregivers page (www.betaseron.com/beta/caregive/patient.jsp). One can also find information on local support groups there or through visiting the organization's home page at www.betaseron.com. A list of organizations hosting support groups provides routes to contact information on the local level. Organizations listed in this section include some of the national groups mentioned above, the International MS Support Foundation, the Consortium of Multiple Sclerosis Centers, and various online support groups.

IN A SENTENCE:

> *MS support groups, which can be a great benefit, are easily located on the Internet or through your local contacts.*

living

Taking Stock

LAST MONTH was a good time to evaluate the major relationships in your life. As you continue treating your MS and
treating yourself well, make the time now to review how you
yourself are doing. Take stock of your feelings about dealing
with the disease and about your life in general. Are you relatively content with your daily life, doing the best you can with
the cards MS has dealt you? Are you subject to wide shifts in
mood, perhaps even consumed at times by anger because of the
unfairness of having MS?

Ask yourself questions like these. If you wish, sit down with
a trusted friend, a minister or rabbi, or a therapist to examine
the answers and discuss their implications.

Finding happiness

Feeling good is a great gift, but happiness doesn't just happen—you have to help make it happen. Having good things to
look forward to helps make for a reasonably happy and productive life. Hope can be good medicine, and even an expectation that is ultimately disappointed will have given you at least
momentary joy. For instance, a friend of mine buys a lottery
ticket every week. When I asked him why he continued to do

this after having been disappointed for years, he responded, "That dollar buys me a week of hope. That's worth it to me."

Laughter is another key to happiness. In his groundbreaking book *Anatomy of an Illness,* Norman Cousins wrote, "I was greatly elated by the discovery that there is a physiologic basis for the ancient theory that laughter is good medicine." If you haven't had a good laugh lately, watch a favorite video, or share a funny story with family or friends. It's a great tonic.

In *The Biology of Hope,* Cousins provides a lot of tips about staying upbeat, using hope and humor to maintain a positive attitude while battling a chronic condition.

The persistence of anger

Anger is an emotion both sexes experience, but it is not gender neutral. Although women diagnosed with MS feel anger—huge amounts in some cases, irrational amounts, and they may rant and rave—it's usually contained and often doesn't affect how they function everywhere else. For example, a woman may be angry but she'll still cook dinner for her family. On the other hand, in the men whom I have spoken with, I found their feelings of anger seemed to come from a sense of emotional impotency.

Take Matthew, for instance, a man who was diagnosed with MS at the age of thirty-two. His wife warned him continually that his bad moods were hurting their three children, and he was neglecting the kids too. Matthew says he believed "I was the only one suffering," but when his wife finally called a family meeting to discuss his long-standing anger, "I got my comeuppance. My family still loved me. That made me know I had to do better. I literally stopped being angry. Just stopped. And started finding ways to help make our family work better, and I regained their trust in me."

Psychologists and feminists can debate whether men and women are inherently different. But I know that my reactions to having MS have been different from those of the men I've spoken to. Generally, there are real differences in the ways most men and most women deal with any understandable continuing bursts of anger about having MS. So let's stop looking at causes here and examine one thing you can do to channel your anger in a more positive direction.

Giving back to others

When you concentrate on helping others, you focus on the task at hand and lose sight of whatever has been preoccupying you. In that light, many people with MS have reported that doing something for somebody else—a family member, a friend, another person with MS, or a more amorphous contribution to the community—is a very effective way to defuse any residual anger. Giving back also bestows on you a sense of accomplishment and self-worth.

The ways in which you make a contribution depend on you and your situation. Some can do more physically than others, and some people have a strong desire to do more. What you offer others may be as simple as a special meal for your family, or bringing flowers home to your spouse or partner. You may choose to devote more uninterrupted time to your children, or help one of them with a homework problem. If you have time and enjoy volunteering, you might work a few hours weekly at your local library or hospital. If there is a community garden near your home, you may help maintain it, for the sake of both the garden and yourself. If you are handy and you knit, crochet, sew, build birdhouses, or have other craft skills, make something for someone you love. No gift is as appreciated as one that is handmade.

Drawing on your professional background is an easy way to volunteer. For example, I am a children's-book writer, and I never turn down a chance to read to young children, whether at public schools, private schools, or libraries. Soon I will be reading to children in foster care as well. Not only am I giving back, I'm getting so much more than I give—kids give themselves, and that's the best.

If you feel up to it and you can afford it, you may want to make an annual pledge to a charity of your choice. By the way, it need not be the National Multiple Sclerosis Society, although this is a logical and positive choice. On a smaller scale, you may want to help start a support group in your area to aid others who are newly diagnosed like yourself, either by helping to initially organize it or by pledging to pay for the rental of meeting space at the beginning.

Helping others, in turn, helps to keep you from becoming so self-absorbed that you become actually selfish. You don't want to get into the situation Matthew did, neglecting those you love because of the funk you find yourself in.

If you are stuck in a funk of anger because of the hand of cards your MS has dealt you, remind yourself that life is unfair. You may feel that life owes you one now, but it doesn't work that way. Don't sit around waiting for life to pay up. Give instead, and you may be able to recall just how much others have and are giving or trying to give to you.

Helping in the MS community

As you accumulate experience with MS, you become a valuable resource for others. Your expertise can help people who are recently diagnosed, who need someone who's been there to share feelings with, or who have never had to cope with a symptom that you are used to. This wisdom you have regarding the disease is one more excellent reason not to try to keep your MS a secret.

One obvious person who gives back is the talk-show host Montel Williams. Another prominent person who gives back is Liane Mark of Honolulu. She was competing in beauty pageants to help pay for her college loans. On the very night she was crowned Miss Waikiki, she felt a tingling in her feet. She attributed it to the amount of time she had spent standing in ridiculously high heels, but it continued, and the rest is history. She was diagnosed with MS at the age of twenty-four. While she did not go on to become Miss America, Liane has gone on to be a great American. Her purpose is to pass on all the hope and inspiration she can to those living with MS.

She began helping others by first volunteering at her local NMSS chapter. Now she travels the country talking at fund-raisers, hospitals, and schools. Among other things, she is adamant about clearing up all kinds of misconceptions about this mystery ailment—from being living proof that MS need not "cripple the young" or make you old to focusing on the nearly 40 percent of those diagnosed with MS who refuse to seek treatment. She is on disease-modifying medication; and, by the way, though she self-injects, when she's just not up to doing it herself, her dad helps.

We can all be grateful for Liane's positive voice and advocacy for better awareness and treatment of MS, and take inspiration from her philosophy of hope, determination, and giving back to others.

Clearly not all of us lead high-profile lives that allow us the opportunity to be interviewed and tell our stories of MS to *People* magazine, as Liane Mark did, but you can give back much closer to home. Carla told me she was waiting in her chiropractor's waiting room and was asked by an older woman sitting next to her why she saw a chiropractor. She explained briefly about her MS. The woman kept asking questions, and Carla answered them openly. The woman then said, "You are a very inspiring person. Are you an inspirational speaker?" Carla said no, but thanked her. She says, "I didn't want to say, I'd never do that in my life. But I kept thinking about it, and eventually I started a support group online that's helping me and everyone else in the group." Giving back can be as simple as that.

IN A SENTENCE:

> *Take stock of where you are in life, and, if you can, start to help others—your family, those with MS, or in your community.*

learning

Trends in
MS Research

MANY INTERESTING treatment possibilities for MS are being examined and tested by researchers. Some of them may become available in the immediate future. This should give us first-year members of the MS club reason for enthusiasm.

However, at the same time, we must understand that there are no miracle cures. What is interesting about so-called sudden breakthroughs in scientific research on MS is just how many years may go into what is considered a sudden breakthrough. I am reminded of the rock star who said upon being told that he was an overnight success, "Thanks. It only took me fifteen years."

Immunology

While the cause of MS remains unknown, many scientists are working on the supposition that an immune-system disorder is the culprit (as was discussed earlier).

When the immune system turns against the body it is designed to protect, it is called an autoimmune disorder. Autoimmunity might be described as a civil war of the body. We know now that this civil war is going on, but scientists may soon discover the cause of this war. At this point, research has already identified errant immune cells, which invade the nervous system (where they do not belong). Now scientists are trying to understand how components of the immune system are transformed into dysfunctional elements that go on to cause autoimmune diseases. This information promises to contribute dramatically to the new and innovative therapies for MS.

The human genome

Genetic research into the causes of MS is a fairly new area of exploration. The mapping of the human genome has already led to a number of startling discoveries, which gives us reason to hope that if there is a gene that causes MS, or predisposes a person toward getting the disease, it will be identified soon. Through genetic analysis it may become possible to determine specific susceptibility to the development of MS within families where the disease has already occurred, as well as within the general population. Being able to tell who is at risk for the disease may help promote early intervention with the new disease-modifying therapies and, thereby, keep disability to a minimum or perhaps even prevent any disability from developing.

Infectious diseases

General agreement among the experts has been reached on the autoimmune nature of MS. But what agent triggers the autoimmune system to turn upon itself? This is where research in the area of infectious disease comes into the picture. For years, the hunt has been on for a viral infection that triggers the onset of MS. Now, the possibility of bacterial infection triggering the onset of the disease is also under scrutiny. The bacterium most examined is *Chlamydia pneumoniae,* which is also known to cause "walking pneumonia." So far, some research has established the presence of this bacterium in MS tissues and in people dealing with MS. But if such a common bacterium is designated as the trigger or cause of MS, then everyone who ever contracted walking pneumonia would theoretically be at risk and, certainly, their incidence of MS would have to be much higher. So far, no one has found such a direct link, which suggests that this bacterium is not the sole trigger for the disease.

A consensus is emerging among researchers that there is probably no one virus, bacterium, or infectious agent related to the development of MS. The focus is shifting to the interaction of an individual's immune system and the invaders it faces.

Stay tuned, as we all will. In addition, if you are a member of a support group and have information regarding an early childhood or teenage illness that laid you low, share it with your group. Pass it on to your doctor as well, and contribute an article about your experience to the publication sponsored by your disease-modifying medication or another magazine you have access to. The information we share may be the cornerstone of future medical investigations and disease-treatment progress.

Glial cells

In addition to neurons, glial cells are a major component of the CNS. It appears that their primary purpose, as they develop in the first stages of cell life, is to form myelin. Research is now focusing on how immune-system responses affect glial cells in their early stages and the early development of myelin, as well as on how the scars of demyelination are registered on them. With much further research, scientists may discover a way to get the glial cells of people with MS to regenerate myelin.

Clinical trials

Clinical trials are often used to test the effectiveness of new medical treatments. The patients enrolled in the study are divided into two groups; both receive the treatment, but whether it is an injection or a pill, one group receives the experimental treatment and the other receives a placebo, a harmless substance packaged to resemble the real medication. The health of all participants is rigorously monitored; in the case of a trial for an MS drug, you would be watched closely for any side effects, relapses, exacerbations, and so on. People in the study do not know which group they are in, and usually the medical professionals administering the medication and performing checkups on you don't know either.

Such trials are possible only with the help of people like us—people who live with MS. They are the best way to test the effectiveness and safety of new treatments for MS. Clinical research also aids in refining the understanding of MS and the development and refinement of new disease-modifying treatments.

Your MS specialist may ask you to be in a clinical trial, or you may be approached through your support group or find a notice of a new trial on an online message board. Discuss the idea of enrolling in a clinical trial with your MS specialist. He or she will help you understand the pros and cons of such serious volunteerism. You may also want to contact your local chapter of the NMSS for further guidance.

Participating in a clinical trial is a good option for anyone who has minimal or no insurance coverage, since there is usually no charge for the medication and the follow-up medical care. However, clinical trials are not for everyone with MS. Since you will not be told whether you are getting the experimental treatment or a placebo, you may feel anxious wondering whether you're getting any help at all, adding to stress levels. If you're being given the placebo (not that you'll know until after the study is complete, if ever), you will be at risk for further symptoms; on the other hand, if you are being given the real medication, you cannot predict how you will react to the new treatment—with both of these disadvantages, keep in mind that at least you will be closely monitored by the doctors performing the study.

Stem cell research and MS

MS is one of the many conditions which stem cell therapies may become successful in treating. As Martha King, editor in chief of *Inside MS,* stated, "Stem cells are a possible source for repair or replacement strategies for MS." The genius of stem cells is that they possess the ability to produce many types of new cells, thus creating brand-new tissue—something that other cell types cannot do. However, King is also quick to explain that while stem cell research already indicates possible successes in the amelioration of the effects of Alzheimer's, Parkinson's, spinal-cord injuries, MS, and more, the ethical issues that surround the source of the stem cells have provoked an ongoing and highly controversial debate on the subject.

In this ethical debate regarding stem cell research, it is the use of fetal or embryonic stem cells that raises the ruckus. These "universal" stem cells have the highest potential to develop into other types of cells, and they are found only in the earliest developmental stages of the fetus, just after fertilization. The problem is that many factions of the population and the politicians who represent them regard the harvesting of stem cells left over in the discarded embryos created by couples' pursuing in vitro fertilization (IVF) feel this use is immoral.

So far, research indicates that treatment with stem cell therapies may be able to replace dead or damaged tissues caused by MS, but there are still so many unknowns regarding how tissue is damaged by MS in the first place that any actual application of stem cell use in MS treatment is still unclear and needs further scrutiny and investigation.

Research into stem cell therapy in MS is in its earliest stages. However, some results show that mice with MS-like disease recovered mobility when treated with stem cells from the brains of adult mice. The injected cells migrated via the blood to the brain where they generated myelin-making cells in the damaged areas. But mice bred in the laboratory do not experience rejection problems common in humans, and how to safely test such a process in humans is still a major unanswered question.

While it would be wonderful to have positive news regarding the progress of stem cell research and other DNA research in the treatment of MS, there is still the possibility that legislation might be passed limiting exploration of this vital field of new treatment possibilities. Thus, unfortunately, the political debate regarding this scientific issue wears on, and we wait with many others for politicians to protect medical research from too much political infighting, so that research can move forward more quickly to discover therapies that will advance the health and health care of all of us and our loved ones.

If you have the energy, you might want to think about contacting your congressperson on this issue. While I couldn't do so immediately after my diagnosis, I now write to my congressman periodically on the subject—if nothing else, it helps me feel good about doing a little something else for the cause and for myself.

In the meantime, many of those who are dealing with secondary-progressive MS have found that a combination of Zocor and Copaxon to be helpful as a maintenance treatment (see the following section).

Exciting news on statins and MS research

There is exciting news regarding the use of statins in the treatment of MS. Statins, such as Zocor and Lipitor, are usually used to lower cholesterol. Over the past few years researchers have begun to discover that these drugs may be effective in the treatment of autoimmune-related illnesses, including MS. Statins seem to work by lowering the number of new lesions in the brain due to MS.

Apparently, statins have the remarkable ability to reduce the actual inflammation that causes nerve cell damage in the first place. In other words, they act on cells prior to the process of demyelination. Thus, statins may offer a means of preventing the actual progress of the disease, if not a way to prevent the disease itself.

This is particularly true when a statin is used in conjunction with Copaxone, one of the disease-modifying treatments for MS. This is particularly intriguing because treatment with Copaxone is effective in only 30 to 35 percent of patients.

In one study presented at a meeting of the American Academy of Neurology in Honolulu in 2003, Zocor was found to decrease brain lesions from MS in twenty-three out of twenty-eight patients. Other studies on both Zocor and and Lipitor used in conjunction with Copaxone are under way at the University of California and other research centers.

This promising new research on the statin group is considered to be one of the major recent breakthroughs in MS research.

At the present time, treatment with Zocor and Copaxone in combination is available only in clinical trials. Studies involving Lipitor and Copaxone have, until recently, been restricted to testing on mice, but now clinical trials are under way on MS patients.

If your results with Copaxone have so far left something to be desired, you might talk to your doctor about entering a clinical trial involving treatment with Zocor and Copaxone.

If you are taking one of these drugs to lower your cholesterol, obviously your MS specialist is aware of this and found it to be safe for you to continue to take it while taking Copaxone. Be aware that the dose one takes to control cholesterol is much much lower than the dose used in treating symptoms of MS. All clinical trials using statins use the highest approved dose of the statin, which is not the dose used for cholesterol control. *Thus, if you have access to Zocor or Lipitor, do not try this combination on your own at home.*

IN A SENTENCE:

Keep current on new research to remain aware of the best treatment options available to you.

Looking Back, Moving On

SOON IT will be a year since you were first diagnosed with MS, and you've come a long way since that momentous day. That wasn't so hard, was it?

Your first-year anniversary of living with MS is a good time to review how well you're doing. Try to look at the larger picture, knowing that on any individual day, you may feel better or worse.

Until such time as there is a known cure for MS, your goal should be to reach the status of **inactive MS**. Doctors use this term for people who have gone five years without a relapse. Even if you have had a rough first year, it's still something you can aim for. The fact is that treating your MS actively and caring for yourself diligently during your first year lays the foundation for continuing in that way in the future, and the longer you do that well, the better your chances of holding MS at bay.

Review your journal

If you have been keeping a journal or a journal file, the end of your first year with MS is a perfect occasion to look back on the changes you've made in your life, your personal health regimen, and your attitude.

You will probably find a few good truths there. First, and most important, while you may feel that your progress has been slow on a day-to-day basis, reviewing your own words will help you gain perspective on just how far you have come in the last twelve months.

In reviewing my own diary, I came across some sentences I wrote to spur myself on. They might help you too.

○ "Any progress is progress." This came from the first month, when I was still undergoing tests and didn't know what the future would bring. Once I had learned to inject myself, I decided this was so simple, yet true, that I keep it in mind always. Now, with the improvement I've experienced since starting treatment, I believe it more than ever.

○ "Do something, not nothing. If you make a mistake and the something you've done isn't working, you can correct it and achieve the result you are after." I made plenty of mistakes and, with help, have corrected many and made much improvement.

○ "Keep it simple." I wrote down this basic piece of advice from a good friend when I was hyperventilating over a minor crisis. I've already mentioned the idea of keeping it simple in this book, but it bears repeating, since human beings (myself included) are notoriously poor listeners when it comes to their own well-being.

Another bonus to reviewing your journal will be noticing how much more balanced your emotional equilibrium has become.

Remind yourself that you are on the right track

As you've gained experience dealing with MS on a day-to-day basis, you may also increasingly find yourself listening to your own instincts about how to handle new situations. And with experience comes wisdom, which helps you put it all in perspective. Use your hard-earned MS wisdom to evaluate whether you're on the right track; keep note of where you've done exceptionally well and where you know you need improvement.

Sometime toward the end of my first year on Avonex, my MS wisdom led me to a new and comforting view of my situation as a person with MS. I was out walking on a cool fall day. I thought about how MS has changed none of the fundamental things in my life: I am getting older; I have the same responsibilities, if not more; the stresses in my life are as great as the stresses in anyone's. Yet, even as I realized this, a voice inside me said, "I don't want to jinx my progress but *I feel better*."

Later, when I sat down to evaluate why it was that I felt better, I could see there were a number of elements that had been working slowly to my benefit. Until I was hit with the revelation, which part of me didn't want to jinx by even thinking about, that I hadn't seen how the little things add up.

Become your own MS expert

Let me tell you one last thing that's happened to me that may have some bearing on how you continue to live with MS. It started late last November, when I fixed a big dinner one Friday night for family and friends. Afterward, I was doing the dishes with a helpful ten-year-old who accidentally dropped a soapy china plate on my right foot. I said nothing about the pain. She felt bad enough. We finished our chores, and the guests went home. By ten my toe was black and blue and the bruise had spread up the foot. I was reluctant to call my doctor over the weekend—after all, this was not a "real" emergency.

When I saw my internist early the next week, he suggested an X-ray, but was not insistent. He knows by now, that after all the procedures I've been through, I'm a bit leery of immediately X-raying every body part because of a mere glancing pain. Instead, I soldiered on, walking on (not working through) my pain.

A few days later, I had another fall, breaking it with my right foot rather than falling face forward and breaking my teeth. Once again, I shrugged and went about my business. It was a busy season—my son's birthday comes right before the December holidays—and the foot seemed like a passing problem, something minor that would resolve itself.

However, pain is there for a reason: it exists to tell you that something is wrong. And I wasn't listening, as I discovered once I finally did make the time (well into the new year) to go in for that X-ray. It turned out I had spent enough time walking on that foot to dislocate the joint in the second toe. I was then given an elastic splint to try to bring the toe back into place before the toes became hammertoes, given a postoperative shoe to wear, and told I would need a cortisone injection. The next day, I called my MS specialist to make sure this would not interfere with my Avonex injection.

It would take my toes and foot a long time to recover. The lessons of this story are twofold.

First, as any of us complete our first year with MS, we feel a solid sense of accomplishment. We count our blessings and, while not gloating or feeling triumphant, we know we have navigated a hard and long year well. But temper the pride you rightly feel with the real wisdom that, like me, you're still capable of making a doozy of a mistake, one that could impact your wellness. Stay vigilant against such slip-ups, and remember to ask for assistance from family and friends when you need it.

Second, I have just guided you through your initial year of MS, helping you learn the medical facts and sharing the tips that have made it easier for me and others with MS to adjust to their new condition. But, as this incident makes clear, I'm not perfect—I make my share of errors and I don't know all the answers. So don't take anything I have said about living with MS as the only way it can be—your own experience and your own instinct count for a lot. Use them, as well as the other resources you've learned about (your medical team, the Internet, the friends and family members you ask for help, and so on) in the best way you can, and continue improving a personal program that works well for you in fighting MS.

Congratulations on having gotten this far, and good luck in becoming your own best MS expert in the years to come!

IN A SENTENCE:

> *Give yourself a big pat on the back for reaching the one-year milestone, and celebrate your life.*

learning

How to Keep Learning—the Internet

IN RECENT years, the Web has virtually exploded in terms of making available megaloads of information. Space does not permit listing every pertinent website for valuable information on MS. The sites suggested here will offer you further choices as you begin your Internet research on MS, and you will very soon become a terrific MS sleuth on your own.

The Internet is your best source to keep learning about MS, finding out about new treatment options as they are approved for the public and staying current on the latest developments on the research front. Once you are Internet-savvy, you can navigate your way regularly to the best websites, those that work as both a positive informational source and a form of emotional support.

In addition to the simplicity of going online in your own home, many people newly diagnosed with MS find the anonymity afforded by MS discussion groups, message boards, and chat rooms to be perfectly designed for their needs.

Here are six organizations whose websites are a good place for you to start in your Internet explorations.

Web MD Health: Multiple Sclerosis Center

www.webmd.com/diseases_and_conditions/multiple_sclerosis.htm

This site gives good general information about multiple sclerosis. It includes a sampling of full-text articles with current information on MS. There are discussions of symptoms and treatment options. There are message boards and live-event transcripts available. The site's interface allows for clear and easy navigation to the resources offered.

Multiple Sclerosis International Federation

www.msif.org

This site, produced in the United Kingdom, is extremely impressive and informative. It offers knowledge on all aspects of the illness, (symptoms, medication, and origin theories presented by professionals) and also sponsors seminars, message boards, and chat rooms. Social aspects of the illness are dealt with, such as how the Internet provides a means for those suffering from MS to connect with one another. This site is very concerned with connecting MS patients into a community of people working to learn, share, and overcome the illness together, from across the globe. A variety of links to other Internet sites about MS are also available.

National Multiple Sclerosis Society

www.nationalmssociety.org

The official site of the NMSS provides new information about MS and treatments for it. This site is also very concerned with rallying people to advocate for a cure for MS—for instance, there's a list of upcoming fund-raising events to benefit the fight against the disease. Information on educational programs is also plentiful.

Consortium of Multiple Sclerosis Centers

www.mscare.org

Besides providing online forums to discuss MS and any related topics, this very professional website serves as a bibliographic source for those seeking MS information. It provides recent lectures and journal articles on MS, as well as information on the most recent books dealing with the disease. Although it's not as extensive a website as some

of the others in this section, the knowledge provided is clearly presented and always professional in nature.

MSWorld
www.msworld.org

 MSWorld is a valuable site for those dealing with MS. It is
designed in such a way that one feels a comfortable and healing
atmosphere when surfing through what the site provides. Much of
the site's content is oriented toward the personal experiences of those
with MS, including how to deal with relationships with spouses,
partners, family, and friends. Chat rooms and message boards are
offered, and new books and articles dealing with living with MS are
reviewed. Much of the material is inspirational in nature.

Multiple Sclerosis: Its Diagnosis, Symptoms, Types, and Stages
http://thjuland.tripod.com/multiple-sclerosis.html
also www.geocities.com/hotsprings/3468/multiple-sclerosis.html

 Created by Dr. Thomas J. Copeland, who has MS, this easily nav-
igable site contains a wide variety of information. It provides a good
introduction to a basic understanding of the illness (some sites can
be overwhelming and too heavy with information). Click on the
"Mscapades" section for a detailed account of Copeland's own experience when first being diagnosed with MS—a long and confusing
process that others may relate to. Helpful links, some bibliographical information, and a glossary of terms are included.

IN A SENTENCE:

> *Never stop learning, and you will never stop growing.*

Glossary

ACTIVE MS: A term used to describe clinically diagnosed MS in which lesions appear on the MRI and the patient has experienced one or more episodes or relapses and has a number of noticeable symptoms.

ANTIBODIES: Proteins of the immune system that reside in blood and other bodily fluid. They are produced to fight invasion by bacteria, viruses, and other outside antigens entering the body. Certain antibodies are more present in people with MS.

AUTOIMMUNE DISEASE: An illness in which the body's immune system mistakenly attacks healthy cells and tissues in the body. Multiple sclerosis is believed to be an autoimmune disease.

AXONS: The nerve fibers that serve as the highways on which electrical signals carrying messages and information are transported throughout the central nervous system. Axons are often damaged by demyelination.

BENIGN MS: In this form of relapsing-remitting multiple sclerosis, accounting for 5 percent of RRMS cases (and just over 1 percent of all cases of MS), you don't get worse over time and there is no permanent disability. Even an MS specialist can't tell that you have this until several years after the episode that led to the initial diagnosis of MS.

CENTRAL NERVOUS SYSTEM (CNS): The section of the nervous system that includes the brain, the optic nerves, and the spinal cord.

DEMYELINATION: A loss of myelin in the nervous system. The loss of myelin causes the development of scar tissue.

EXACERBATION: The appearance of new symptoms or the worsening of old ones. Exacerbation is usually the result of inflammation or demyelination in either the brain or along the spinal cord.

IMD: See Intramuscular deep injection.

INACTIVE MS: A term used to describe clinically diagnosed MS in which lesions appear on the MRI, but the person has not experienced a relapse for at least five years.

INTERFERON: Substances produced by the body's immune system in response to viral infections. There are several kinds of interferon. Interferon beta-1a and Interferon beta-1b have been approved for use in ambulatory individuals with relapsing-remitting MS. These drugs reduce the frequency of exacerbations.

INTRAMUSCULAR DEEP INJECTION (IMD): A method of administering disease-modifying medications. Using a 1½-inch needle, the drug is injected deep into the muscle.

MAGNETIC RESONANCE IMAGING (MRI): A diagnostic method of producing visual images of the body without the use of X-rays. An MRI makes it possible to visualize and count lesions in the white matter of the brain and spinal cord. Also referred to as nuclear magnetic resonance (NMR).

MRI: See Magnetic Resonance Imaging.

MYELIN: A coating of nerve fibers in the central nervous system composed of lipids and protein. Myelin is an aid to nerve fiber protection and sensory conduction. When it is damaged, as can happen with multiple sclerosis, nerve fiber conduction may become faulty or fail.

MYELIN BASIC PROTEIN: A protein that makes up approximately 30 percent of myelin. This protein can often be found in higher than normal concentrations in the cerebrospinal fluid of individuals with MS. One theory is that myelin basic protein is an antigen that triggers autoimmune responses in people with MS.

PLAQUE: A section of inflamed or demyelinated central nervous system tissue.

PRIMARY-PROGRESSIVE MS: A course of MS characterized by a progressive steady decline, with either no or very short-lived plateaus and remissions. About 15 percent of people with MS have primary-progressive MS.

PROGRESSIVE-RELAPSING MS: A severe variety of MS, accounting for 3 percent of cases. This complex form of the disease, which calls for aggressive treatment, is also called Marburg MS.

RELAPSE: A period when symptoms of MS that you've had in the past recur to an aggravated degree and for a longer period of time. Relapses are sometimes referred to as incidents, attacks, or episodes.

RELAPSING-REMITTING MS (RRMS): A type of MS characterized by occasional relapses, followed by a full or partial recovery and then a period when the disease seems in remission. About 42 percent of people with MS have RRMS.

REMISSION: A period when symptoms lessen in severity or disappear altogether.

REMYELINATION: The repair of damaged myelin. In individuals with MS, remyelination occurs very slowly.

SECONDARY-PROGRESSIVE MS: The second most common type of MS, accounting for 40 percent of cases, it develops after relapsing-remitting

MS. After a period, often five to twenty years, when a person has RRMS, there is an overall worsening of the person's condition, including more frequent relapses and less complete remissions, and the disease is reclassified as secondary-progressive.

SIGNS: Evidence of the disease that the doctor sees for him- or herself during an examination. Signs of MS include overactive reflexes, vision disorders, weakness in specific limbs, and abnormal patterns of speech.

SILENT MS: Also referred to as invisible MS, this is a type of the disease that has been very hard to identify and diagnose, since there are no visible external symptoms. However, a person with silent MS does have lesions on the brain, which would be seen on an MRI.

SPASTICITY: An abnormal increase in muscle tone, resulting in the springlike resistance of a limb or other extremity to moving or being moved.

SUBCUTANEOUS INJECTION (SI): A method of administering disease-modifying medications. The drug is injected just beneath the skin, via a ¾-inch needle.

SYMPTOMS: Physical manifestations, suggesting something is wrong, that a patient reports to a doctor. Symptoms of MS include fatigue, spasticity, vertigo, tremor, and weakness.

VERTIGO: A dizzy, spinning sensation that can be accompanied by nausea or, in extreme cases, vomiting.

For Further Reading

Bowling, Allen C., M.D., Ph.D. *Alternative Medicine and Multiple Sclerosis.* New York: Demos Medical Publishing, 2001.

Carroll, David L., and Jon Dudley Dorman, M.D. *Living Well with MS: A Guide for Patient, Caregiver, and Family.* New York: HarperCollins, 1993.

Cooper, Laura D. *Insurance Solutions—Plan Well, Live Better: A Workbook for People with a Chronic Disease or Disability.* New York: Demos Medical Publishing, 2001.

Cousins, Norman: *Anatomy of an Illness as Perceived by the Patient.* New York: Bantam, 1995.

Eades, Michael, M.D., and Mary Dan Eades, M.D. *Protein Power.* New York: Bantam, 1996.

Fortgang, Laura Berman. *Living Your Best Life.* New York: Tarcher/Putnam, 2001.

Garr, Teri. *Speedbumps: Flooring It Through Hollywood.* New York: Hudson Street Press, 2005.

Graham, Judy. *Multiple Sclerosis: A Self-Help Guide to Its Management.* Rochester, Vt.: Healing Arts Press, 1989.

Hill, Beth Ann. *Multiple Sclerosis Q & A: Reassuring Answers to Frequently Asked Questions.* New York: Avery, 2003.

Holland, Nancy J., T. Jock Murray, and Stephen C. Reingold. *Multiple Sclerosis: A Guide for the Newly Diagnosed.* 2nd ed. New York: Demos, 2002.

Klug, Michael J., M.D., ed. *Johns Hopkins Family Health Book.* New York: HarperCollins, 1999.

Larson, David E., M.D., ed. *The Mayo Clinic Family Health Book.* New York: William Morrow, 1990.

Lechtenberg, Richard, M.D., F.A. *Multiple Sclerosis Fact Book*. Philadelphia: Davis Company, 1995.

Mosby's Pocket Dictionary of Medicine, Nursing, and Allied Health. 2nd ed. St. Louis: Mosby, 1994.

Myss, Caroline, Ph.D. *Anatomy of the Spirit: The Seven Stages of Power and Healing*. New York: Crown, 1996.

Nichols, Judith Lynn, and Her Online Group of MS Sisters. *Women Living with Multiple Sclerosis*. Berkeley, Calif.: Hunter House, 1999.

Reeve, Christopher. *Nothing Is Impossible: Reflections on a New Life*. New York: Ballantine, 2004.

Rogers, Judy, and Molleen Matsumura. *The Disabled Woman's Guide to Pregnancy and Birth*. New York, Demos Medical Publishing, 2006.

Rosner, Louis J., M.D., and Shelley Ross. *Multiple Sclerosis: New Hope and Practical Advice for People with MS and Their Families*. Rev. ed. New York: Fireside/Simon & Schuster, 1993.

Russell, Margot, ed. *When the Road Turns: Inspirational Stories by and about People with MS*. Deerfield Beach, Fla.: Health Communications, 2001.

Schapiro, Randall T., M.D. *Symptom Management in Multiple Sclerosis*. 3rd ed. New York: Demos, 1998.

Schwarz, Shelley Peterman. *Multiple Sclerosis: 300 Tips for Making Life Easier*. New York: Demos Medical Publishing, 2006.

Shernoff, William M. *Fight Back and Win: How to Get Your HMO and Health Insurance to Pay Up*. Sterling, VA: Capital Books, 1999.

Taub, Edward A., M.D. *The Wellness Rx*. Englewood Cliffs, N.J.: Prentice Hall, 1994.

Weil, Andrew, M.D. *Spontaneous Healing*. New York: Fawcett Columbine, 1995.

Weil, Andrew, M.D., and Rosie Daley. *The Healthy Kitchen: Recipes for a Better Body, Life, and Spirit*. New York: Knopf, 2002.

MULTIPLE SCLEROSIS ORGANIZATIONS

National Multiple Sclerosis Society
(NMSS)
733 Third Avenue, 3rd Floor
New York, NY 10017
800-FIGHT-MS (800-344-4867)
www.nationalmssociety.org
E-mail: info@nmss.org
> Besides providing information you need regarding insurance, the NMSS can put you in touch with a local chapter in your area.

DISABILITY IN GENERAL

Accent on Information
P.O. Box 700
Bloomington, IL 61702
304-378-2961
> Accent on Information is a computerized system that retrieves information for the disabled concerning difficulties connected to activities of daily life and personal management. There is a small fee for the use of this service, but people with disabilities are never denied this service if they are unable to pay.

jjMarketing Inc
1205 Savoy Street, Suite 101
San Diego, CA 92107
619-222-8735
Fax: 619-226-2675

Descriptive Video Service (DVS)
125 Western Avenue
WGBH
Boston, MA 02134
800-333-1203
317-579-0439 (to rent videos; available 24 hours a day)
E-mail: access@wgbh.org
www.wgbh.org/dvs/
> DVS's services are extremely helpful to those with vision problems. Write to obtain quarterly information on movies and programs being offered in the DVS Guide.

Easter Seals Canada
90 Eglinton Avenue East, Suite 208
Toronto, Ontario M4P 2Y3
Canada
416-932-8383
www.easterseals.ca
info@easterseals.ca
  This organization is a federation of
  groups serving people with disabilities
  throughout Canada.

Canadian Rehabilitation Council for the
  Disabled (CRCD)
65 Brunswick St.
Frederickton, NB E3B 1G5
Canada
506-458-8739
www.sjfn.nb.ca

Health Resource Center for Women with
  Disabilities
Rehabilitation Institute of Chicago
Chicago, IL 60612
312-238-1051

National Council on Disability
1331 F Street NW, Suite 850
Washington, D.C. 20004-1107
www.ncd.gov

Paralyzed Veterans of America (PVA)
801 18th Street, NW
Washington D.C. 20006
202-USA-1300
800-424-8200
www.pva.org
  Among other services, PVA provides
  assistance to U.S. veterans diagnosed
  with MS.
  Healthcare Hotline: 800-232-1782

National Rehabilitation Information Center
  (NARIC)
4200 Forbes Boulevard, Suite 202
Lanham, MD 20706
800-346-2742
Fax: 301-459-4263
www.naric.com

Social Security Administration
800-772-1213 (7:00 A.M. to 7:00 P.M.,
Monday through Friday, Eastern time)
  Ask for "Disability Benefits," a pam-
  phlet outlining what an applicant for
  Social Security benefits may be eligible for. You can request a Social
  Security application, an estimate of
  what your benefits may be if you have
  an employment history, and other
  information from this same number.

United Spinal Association
75-20 Astoria Boulevard
Jackson Heights, NY 11370
718-803-EPVA
www.unitedspinal.com
  Provides help to U.S. veterans in the
  eastern portion of the country, as
  well as providing information outreach
  services.

Well Spouse Foundation
63 West Main Street, Suite H
Freehold, NJ 07728
800-838-0879
www.wellspouse.org

COMPLEMENTARY AND ALTERNATIVE MEDICINE

American Apitherapy Society
5535 Balboa Boulevard, Suite 225
Encino, CA 91316
818-501-0446
www.apitherapy.org
  For information on bee venom therapy
  (BVM).

American Academy of Medical
  Acupuncture
4929 Wilshire Boulevard, Suite 428
Los Angeles, CA 90010
323-937-5514
www.medicalacupuncture.org

American Association of Oriental
  Medicine
PO Box 162349
Sacramento, CA 95816
916-443-4770 or 866-455-7999
  (toll free)
www.aaom.org

American Chiropractic Association
1701 Clarendon Boulevard
Arlington, VA 22209
703-276-8800 or 800-986-4636
www.amerchiro.org

American Hippotherapy Association
136 Bush Road
Damascus, PA 18415
888–851–4592
www.americanhippotherapyassociation.com

American Massage Therapy Association
500 Davis Street, Suite 900
Evanston, IL 60201-4695
877–905–2700
www.amtamassage.org

International Institute of Reflexology
5650 First Avenue North
P.O. Box 12642
St. Petersburg, FL 33733
727-343-4811
www.reflexology-usa.net

National Center for Homeopathy (NCH)
801 North Fairfax Street, Suite 306
Alexandria, VA 22314
703-548-7790
www.homeopathic.org

National Certification Board for
    Therapeutic Massage and Bodywork
1901 S. Meyers Road, Suite 240
Oakbrook Terrace, IL 60181
800-296-0664
www.ncbtmb.com

EMPLOYMENT AND LABOR LAW
Equal Employment Opportunity
    Commission
1801 L Street, NW, 10th Floor
Washington, DC 20507
800-669-4000
www.eeoc.gov

EMPLOYMENT AND LABOR LAW
C. O. Bigelow Chemists
414 Avenue of the Americas
New York, NY 10011
212-533-2700 (general) or 212-982-
7580 (surgical supply department)
or 800–793–5433
www.bigelowchemists.com
    The oldest apothecary in the United
    States, Bigelow will ship anywhere in
    the United States. The store has an
    extensive surgical supply department, it
    has the disease-modifying medications
    in stock (many pharmacies have to spe-
    cial-order it), and it also carries a com-
    plete range of homeopathic remedies.

Institute Fulfillment Center
c/o The Cost Containment Research
    Institute
4200 Wisconscin Avenue NW,
    Suite 106–222
Washington, DC 20016
202–318–0770
    If you have financial concerns that
    make MS treatment prohibitively
    expensive, this organization has infor-
    mation that can help you. It publishes a
    free pamphlet, "Free and Low Cost
    Drugs" (item PD-370), which is avail-
    able in a printed version or, an elec-
    tronic version online.

The Medicine Program
P.O. Box 515
Doniphan, MO 63935-0515
573-996-7300
www.themedicineprogram.com
    Provides a list of company programs
    that contribute drugs to physicians
    treating patients who could not other-
    wise afford medication.

MS Active Source
800-456-2255 (8:30 A.M. to 8:00 P.M.,
Eastern time)
www.MSActiveSource.com
    For information on Avonex.

MS Pathways
800-788-1467 (24 hours a day)
www.mspathways.com
For information on Betaseron.

NeedyMeds
PO Box 63716
Philadelphia, PA 19147
www.needymeds.com
For information on drug-company programs to assist you in obtaining medication.

Pharmaceutical Research and Manufacturers of America (PhRMA)
202-835-3400
www.phrma.org

Shared Solutions
800-887-8100 (Monday through Friday, 8:00 A.M. to 8:00 P.M., Central time)
www.copaxone.com or www.sharedsolutions.com
For information on Copaxone.

INSURANCE AND FINANCE

MSActiveSource
800-456-2255 (8:30 A.M. to 8:00 P.M., Eastern time)
www.msactivesource.com
Members are eligible to consult with a reimbursement specialist concerning insurance claims.

TRAVEL

Access-Able Travel Source (AATS)
P.O. Box 1796
Wheat Ridge, CO 80034
303-232-2929
www.access-able.com
Information on traveling with disabilities.

Society for the Advancement of Travel for the Handicapped (SATH)
347 Fifth Avenue, Suite 610
New York, NY 10016
212-447-7284
www.sath.org
Provides accessible tourism information for disabled travelers, and about promoting travel for the handicapped.

Travelin' Talk
P.O. Box 3534
Clarksville, TN 37043-3534
931-552-6670
www.travelintalk.net

Wilderness Inquiry
808 14th Avenue S.E.
Minneapolis, MN 55414
800-728-0719
www.wildernessinquiry.org
Wilderness Inquiry organizes trips into the wilderness for people with disabilities, including individuals with MS.

TEENAGERS AND CHILDREN

Teens Inside MS
c/o National Multiple Sclerosis Society
733 Third Avenue, 3rd Floor
New York, NY 10017
800-FIGHT-MS (800–344–4867)
E-mail: info@nmss.org
A great magazine for teens dealing with MS.

MSWorld Chat Room
A chat room on MSWorld designed for teens with MS open to kids ages 13–18 every Thursday starting at 7:00 P.M. Eastern time. To participate, teenagers have to register with MSWorld first and be pre-approved by the moderator. To register, go to www.msworld.org, click on Chat, then click on Register, and follow the instructions from there.

At Our House: a coloring book for children ages 3–5

Someone You Know Has MS: A Book for Families: for ages 6–12

When a Parent Has MS: A Teenager's Guide

Plaintalk: A Booklet About MS for Families
These helpful books, geared toward kids of various ages in families where a parent has been diagnosed with MS, are available from the National Multiple Sclerosis Society.

Parenting with a Disability
c/o Through the Looking Glass
2198 Sixth Street, Suite 100
Berkeley, CA 94710
800–644–2666
www.lookingglass.org
This free quarterly newsletter is just one of many helpful resources Through the Looking Glass offers about coping with disability.

OTHER
National Association of Professional Organizers (NAPO)
4700 W. Lake Avenue
Glenview, IL 60025
847–375–4746
Fax: 877–734–8668
E-mail: hq@napo.net
www.napo.net/about_napo/

Acknowledgments

MY DEEPEST thanks and gratitude to Saud Sadiq, who
is a great person, a great and dedicated doctor, and a man who
gives everything to help others and to change the future for
those who struggle with MS.

I would like to thank all of those living with MS who gave
their time and ideas generously to help me write this informed
book. Special thanks, in particular, are due to Sara Abalan,
Sydney Lewis, and Jack McCrae, who provided much invaluable information on our mutually shared but differently experienced condition. Thanks to Mary Harmon, who has given me
so much help regarding dealing with MS, the writing business,
and the heart of it all—helping each other. Thanks, Mary.

My profound thanks also to the other dedicated and wonderful doctors who help me all the time: Ludmilla Bronfin, Dena
Harris, Jeffrey Larken, Frank Lipman, Kate Sadowska, Marc
Siegel, and Carol Zietz, all great doctors and people, and to Ruby
and the rest of the team at Avonex Direct Delivery and Nova
Factor who always got me my medicine on time and thanks now
to Caremark Pharmacy who do the same for me under my new
insurance coverage. My love and appreciation to my friend Jenny

Doctorow, who started me on my journey toward finding the best doctors for me in the world.

Gratitude is also due to my agent, Joelle Delbourgo, who thought of me immediately for the project and gave me confidence and inspiration all along the way. And to Trent Duffy, friend and consummate artist when it comes to book editing and organizing.

In addition, great thanks and gratitude goes to my publisher and editor, Matthew Lore. Thanks also to Sue McCloskey, his associate editor, the rest of the Marlowe staff, and particularly to designers Howard Grossman and Pauline Neuwirth.

Immense gratitude goes to my editor, Renée Sedliar, who made me feel how important this revised edition was, gave me too many (much appreciated) compliments, and was unstinting in giving her encouragement and time and expert editorial eye to every word I wrote. I owe her all my thanks and more; thanks also to her great intern Emily Schneider, who did hands-on work on the project.

Thanks forever to my son, Dashiell Lunde, who motivates and inspires me, and makes me so proud. Thanks for always being a better speller than I am and for being willing to shout out the spelling of a word I can't correct by spell-check.

Thanks always to my mom, Barbara Blackstone, great brain, great dame, who actually got me involved in the National Multiple Sclerosis Society. Her friend, Gloria Hammond, started sending me the NMSS magazine. Great friend, great magazine.

Thanks to the National Multiple Sclerosis Society, in particular thanks to Martha King, editor of *Inside MS,* a great champion of all of us who deal with MS and of doing all that is possible to facilitate new care options of all kinds to those who deal with MS. Thanks also to Thor Hansen, a former director; Nancy Hammond, director of clinical research at the society; and Dorothy Northrop, MSW, ACSW.

Thanks to Jackie Brown, trouper; Felicia de Chabris; Eve Crenovich and her staff at Out of the Kitchen, who kept me and my son in the best sandwiches (for him) and salads (for me), when I had little time; to Pippa Gerrard, who makes me feel important even if I'm not; to Dennis Dalrymple and Jamie Raab; to Susan Allison, for her consummate tolerance and grace and good advice and friendship; to Gerardo Alvirez, my personal trainer/physical therapist, who's made me healthier in body and therefore in mind, and is a true friend; and to Channa Taub, who'd like you to think she doesn't have a great big heart, but can't hide it. Thanks to my great friend and neighbor, Claudia Ganz. Also, my great thanks and love go to Michael Simonson, who helped me on the first edition and this new edition in so many ways and, most of all, helped me find my practical bearings in managing my new life with MS. I am lucky to have great friends.

Lastly, I must thank my Newfoundland dog, Lily Louise, who's a few years older but just as dedicated to me getting my work done. She just can't sleep by my feet any longer. Being older and wiser, she needs more space. Let this be a lesson for all of us!